# Handbook of Neurological Physical Therapy

Evidence-Based Practice

**P Shanmuga Raju,** MPT, MIAP

*Head*
Department of Physical Therapy
Chalmeda Anand Rao Institute of Medical Sciences
Karimnagar (Andhra Pradesh)
India

Foreword

C Lakshmi Narasimha Rao
V Surya Narayana Reddy

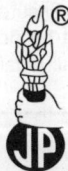

**JAYPEE BROTHERS MEDICAL PUBLISHERS (P) LTD**
New Delhi • Panama City • London

Published by

**Jaypee Brothers Medical Publishers (P) Ltd**

*Corporate Office*

4838/24, Ansari Road, Daryaganj, **New Delhi** 110 002, India
Phone: +91-11-43574357, Fax: +91-11-43574314
Website: www.jaypeebrothers.com

*Offices in India*

- **Ahmedabad**, e-mail: ahmedabad@jaypeebrothers.com
- **Bengaluru**, e-mail: bangalore@jaypeebrothers.com
- **Chennai**, e-mail: chennai@jaypeebrothers.com
- **Delhi**, e-mail: jaypee@jaypeebrothers.com
- **Hyderabad**, e-mail: hyderabad@jaypeebrothers.com
- **Kochi**, e-mail: kochi@jaypeebrothers.com
- **Kolkata**, e-mail: kolkata@jaypeebrothers.com
- **Lucknow**, e-mail: lucknow@jaypeebrothers.com
- **Mumbai**, e-mail: mumbai@jaypeebrothers.com
- **Nagpur**, e-mail: nagpur@jaypeebrothers.com

*Overseas Offices*

- **Central America Office, Panama City, Panama**, Ph: 001-507-317-0160
  e-mail: cservice@jphmedical.com, Website: www.jphmedical.com
- **Europe Office, UK**, Ph: +44 (0) 2031708910
  e-mail: info@jpmedpub.com

*Handbook of Neurological Physical Therapyñ Evidence-Based Practice*

© 2012, Jaypee Brothers Medical Publishers

*First Edition:* 2012

ISBN 978-93-5025-553-7

*Typeset at* JPBMP typesetting unit

*Printed at* Rajkamal Electric Press, Plot No. 2, Phase-IV, Kundli, Haryana.

**To**

**All our Patients at**
*Chalmeda Anand Rao Institute of*
*Medical Sciences Karimnagar*

# Foreword

I am happy to know that Dr P Shanmuga Raju, HOD, Department of Physical Therapy of this Chalmeda Anand Rao Institute of Medical Sciences, Karimnagar, Andhra Pradesh, India is bringing out *Handbook of Neurological Physical Therapy—Evidence Based Practice.*

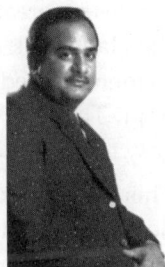

I have gone through the book and found exemplary hard work and interest shown by Dr P Shanmuga Raju in treating the people suffering from various disabilities in the rural areas, where this Institute is located. Neurological disabilities cripple one's life. Overcoming this by Physical Therapy is challenging and Rehabilitation is of utmost concern.

I congratulate Dr P Shanmuga Raju for successfully bringing out this edition. This book would be much help to upcoming physical therapists, faculty, students and all health care professionals.

**C Lakshmi Narasimha Rao** BE MBA
Chairman,
Chalmeda Anand Rao
Institute of Medical Sciences
Arihant Educational Society
Karimnagar
India

# Foreword

It gives me great pleasure to write this foreword for the Handbook of Neurological Physical Therapy Evidence based Practice written by Dr Shanmuga Raju. This book follows a simple principle, and easy to implement it in a day-to-day practice.

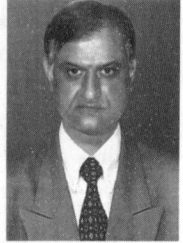

This Handbook explains the problem of threating neurological disability with Physical Therapy interventions in the step by step manner. It is designed to give advance informative, resources and practical guidance for Undergraduate and Postgraduate Physical threapy students and also for the practicing all Rehabilitation professionals. All Chapters dealt with technological interface are equality informative.

I congratulate Dr P Shanmuga Raju for successful completion of this work. I hope that this book will be useful to students and post-graduates.

I wish this book a great success.

**V Surya Narayana Reddy** MS (GEN. SURG)
Director
Chalmeda Anand Rao Institute of
Medical Sciences
Karimnagar, Andhra Pradesh
India

# Preface

*Handbook of Neurological Physical Therapy - Evidence-based Practice*, is to help clinicians make better decisions about patient care. This book is to provide simple format, evidence based Physical Therapy and Rehabilitation.

## Mission

This edition, will be useful to Physical Therapy students, Interns, Medical students, Faculty, Nurse practitioners, Occupational therapists, Physiatrist and physicians Assistant's will find the descriptions of diagnostic and Physical therapy management with citations to the current literature useful in day-to-day patient care.

## Outstanding Features

- Concise, clear presentation of the latest scientific facts, models and methods of practice.
- More than 93 Indian Patients clinical photo gallery.
- Details presentation of all chapters including Neurological examination, Neuroradiology imaging, Physical therapy in Bell's palsy, Stroke physical therapy, Parkinson's disease, Spinal cord injury Rehabilitation, Cerebral palsy, Cerebellar ataxia, and Orthotics in neurological Rehabilitation.
- Recent references, articles, abstracts, and full further editions in writing or via electronic e-mail. The author e-mail address: shanmugampt@rediffmail.com

P Shanmuga Raju

# Acknowledgments

I would like to thank our parents Shri K Perumal, Smt P Nallammal, sisters, and all my teachers.

I express deep thanks to our Chief Patron Shri C Anand Rao, BL, Ex. Minister of law, AP and Social worker, Dr V Bhoom Reddy, MS (AIIMS), Ex-Vice President of National IMA, Shri C Lakshmi Narasimha Rao, BE, MBA, Chairman, Prof. Dr V Surya Narayana Reddy, MS, Director, Arihant Educational Society, Karimnagar, who provided me heart felt support always, in publishing this educational hand book.

My Sincere thanks to Prof. Dr SA Aasim MD, Medical Superintendent, Prnicipal, Prof. Dr Sudha Deshpande, MD, Prof. Dr Jawhar, MS, Prof. Dr Gopal Rao S Jogdand, Ph.D, Prof. Dr N Samanta, M.Ch, Prof. Vittal Reddy, MD, Prof. Dr Aruna, MD, Prof. Dr Neelee Jayasree, MD, Dr Ezhilarasi Ravindhran, MD, Dr. Charan Paul, MD, Dr Jyothi, DGO Dr EV Sridher, MD, Dr Harsha Varadhan, MD, and Mr P Ramakrishana, Mr G Malla Reddy (Steno), Mr Y Venkateshwer Rao, Mr Tiwari, Mr CH Prithvidhar Rao and all CAIMS teaching and nonteaching staff.

I would like to express my thanks to Dr George Williams PT, Dr Hendry Mohan Doss, PT, Prof. Dr V Murugesan, MPT, Prof. Dr SD Sivaganesa, MPT and my friends for their extensive guidance.

I am very grateful to Shri Jitendar P Vij, Group Chairman and CEO, Mr Tarun Duneja, Director (Publishing), Mr Jayanandan, Author Co-ordinator (Chennai), Jaypee Brother's Medical Publishers (P) Ltd, New Delhi, for ideas and extended cooperation in publishing this handbook.

Finally, I thank our patients for their role in inspiring me to write this book.

P Shanmuga Raju

# Contents

# Contents

# Chapter

///////////////////////////////////////

# 1

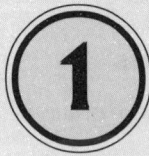

# Neurological Examination

## NEUROLOGICAL EXAMINATION

The Neurological Examination as commonly done includes the important elements such as the mental status, cranial nerves, motor and sensory reflexes, cerebellar function, coordination, gait and station, and other signs.

## HISTORY TAKING AND EXAMINATION

- Patients presenting complaint
- Name, age, sex and exact details of occupation.

### History of Present Illness

- Onset, progression, nature of injury
- Duration
- Mental History
  - Sleep disturbance
  - Speech disturbance
  - Loss of consciousness
  - Headache:
    a. Severity, duration
    b. Tenderness of the scalp or skull
  - Visual disturbance
  - Vomiting and vertigo.
  - History of syphilis
  - Impairment of senses, taste/smell
  - Giddiness
- Movements and sensibility
  - Complaints of muscular weakness
  - Sensory disturbance, especially pain, numbness or tingling
- Abnormal gait
- Sphincters and reproductive function
  - Disturbance of sphincter control
- Nutrition: Weight (stationary, diminishing, increasing).

### Past Medical History

- Surgeries, health factors and other diagnosis.

## Social History

- Occupational and educational history/life style
- Personal habits (tobacco, alcohol).

## Family History

- The family history is often of great importance
- Since many disorders of the central nervous system are hereditary
- The number of children and the occurrence of miscarriage and still births should be assessed.

## Examination of Consciousness (Figs 1.1 and 1.2)

- Is the patient conscious?
- Assess response to stimuli—Glasgow coma scale (GCS)
- No response
- Verbal, tactile, simple commands
- Painful stimuli—Pinching the skin, Pin prick.

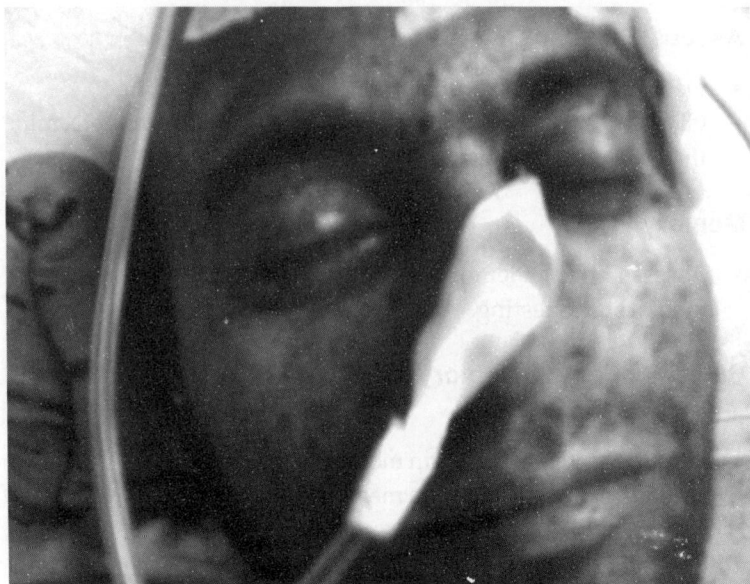

**Fig. 1.1:** Unconsciousness (prior to treatment)

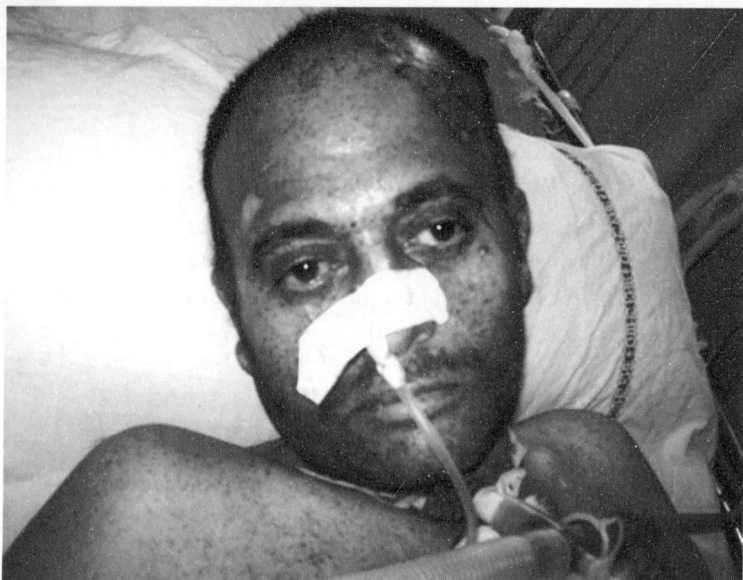

**Fig. 1.2:** Conscious (post-treatment)

## Assess Behavior

- Determine level of confusion, stupor, coma, delirium
- Glasgow Coma Scale (GCS): This scale is utilized to determine the level of consciousness.

## Memory

- Assessment of memory is the most important component of mental status testing.

## Classification of Memory

- Immediate memory
- Recent memory (short-term memory)
- Remote memory (long-term memory).

### Immediate Memory

- Is a very short function?

- Test the patients to remember events such as name, date, week (i.e. 5 minutes).

### Recent Memory

- The patient to recall of recent information such as her address, phone number, and how to come to the present building.

### Remote Memory

- Memory of past events, i.e. birth dates of their children and grand children, where did they grow up.

## Attention

- Assess length of attention span, i.e. digit span retention test, recall of up to 7 members in order presented.
- Assess time on task, frequency of redirection.

## Emotional Response

- The patient is anxious, excited, depressed, frightened, apathetic or euphoric.

## Speech and Communication

- Assess fluency of speech, speech production
- Non fluent aphasia, verbal apraxia
- Dysarthria
- Assess comprehension
  - Aphasia (Fluent), Global (Aphasia).
- Assess nonverbal communication
  - Assess response to use of gestures, symbols, pictographs.

## ASSESS CRANIAL NERVES

1. Cranial nerve I: Olfactory nerve
   - Assess any change in sense of smell and to identify various smells, e.g. deodorants, perfumes, fruits, and soap.
2. Cranial nerve II: Optic nerve
   - Test patient's visual acuity.

- Ask patients to read small print by near vision, and large print at a distance.
3. Cranial nerve III, IV, VI ( Oculomotor, Trochlear and Abducens nerve)
    - III cranial nerve is innervated to superior rectus, medial rectus, inferior rectus, and inferior oblique
    - Assess ptosis: Dropping of the upper eyelid
    - Assess eye movements/note any deviation, asymmetries
    - VI cranial nerve assess pupillary light reflex
    - Test for accommodation.
4. Cranial nerve V Trigeminal nerve:
    - Motor/sensory function
    - Test for Corneal Reflex: Touch cornea with cotton WISP; if absent or dimenshed indicates danger of corneal injuries.
    - Test the jaw jerk by gently tapping your finger placed across the patient's chin with the patella of hammer (Motor function)
    - Assess sensory function (forehead, cheeks, chin).
5. Cranial nerve VII:  Facial nerve
    - Facial expression (wrinkle forehead, show teeth, close eye tightly, puff cheeks) (Figs 1.3 and 1.4)
    - Assess Loss of sensation to anterior 2/3rd of tongue.

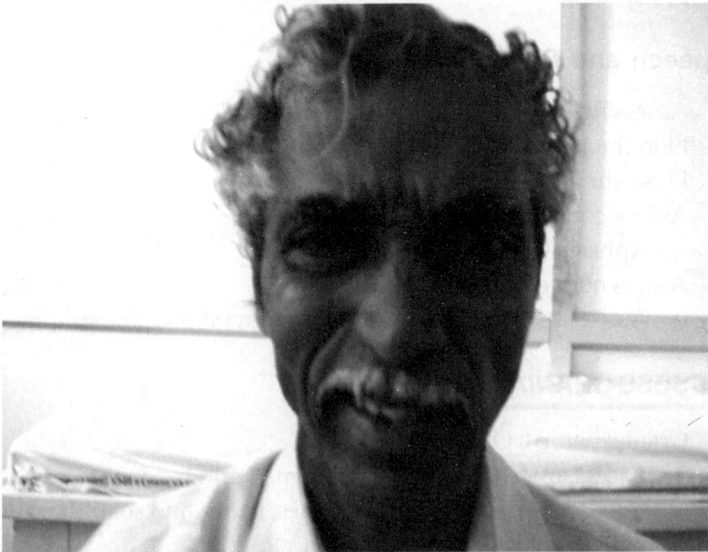

**Fig. 1.3:** Facial (Bell's) paralysis

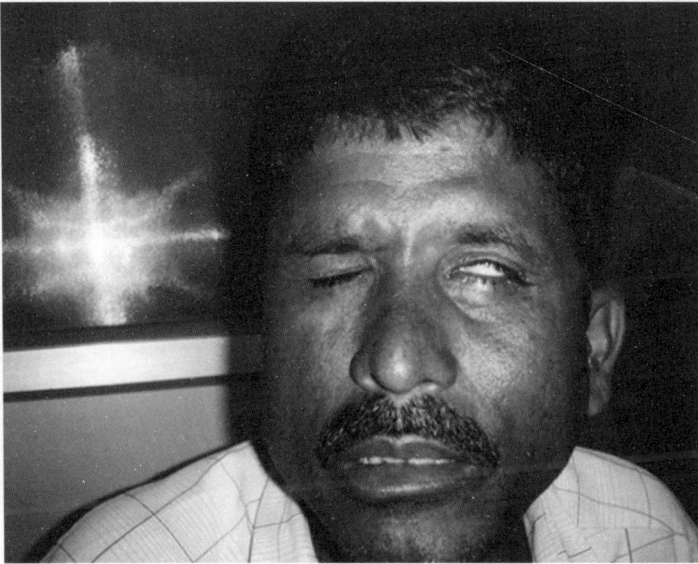

**Fig. 1.4:** Unable to close left eye-ball muscles.

6. Cranial nerve VIII: Vestibulocochlear nerve
   • Assess the external auditory meatus
   • Rhinne's Test: Patient from a tunning fork held close to the ear (air conduction) with the noise heard from a tunning fork placed on the mastoid bone
   • Check hearing acuity
   • Weber's Test: A tuning fork placed on the center of the forehead is normally heard loudest in the deaf ear
   • Help to distinguish between unilateral conductive and perceptive nerve deafness
   • Cranial nerve VIII, Assess balance, posture, vestibular oculat reflex, e.g. nystagmus (involuntary cyclical movements of the eye).
7. Cranial nerve IX: Glosopharyngeal nerve
   • Assess sensory from the posterior 1/3 of tongue.
8. Cranial nerve X: Vagus nerve
   • Assess phonation, articulation. Patient says "Aah"—a unilateral palatal palsy.
   • Assess gag reflex, swallowing.

9. Cranial nerve XI: Spinal Accessory nerve
   - Test the strength of strenoclediomastoid and trapezius muscles.
10. Cranial nerve XII: Hypoglossal nerve
    - Motor nerve
    - Ask the patient to protrude the tongue, note direction, any deviation of movement.
    - Assess power of tongue movements.

## Examination of Vital Signs

1. Heart rate—rhythm, rate.
2. Blood pressure—120/80 mm Hg
   - Hypertension (above 140/100 mm Hg)
   - Hypotension (below 100/60 mm Hg).
3. Respiration—depth, rate, rhythm.
4. Temperature.
5. Pulse.
6. Patttern of breathing
- Cheyne - Stokes Respiration
  - Due to an abnormally increased ventilatory response to $CO_2$ followed post hyperventilation apnea
  - Bilateral cerebral lesions, high brain stem lesion, cardiac disease.
- Sustained deep breathing
  - Midbrain lesions. e.g. tumors, infarction, compression due to herniation
- Irregular breathing
  - Clustered breathing, gasping, or jerking inspiration
  - Medullary lesions
  - Indicating disturbance of the medullary inspiratory and expiratory neurons.

## Check the Vital Signs of CNS

- Nuchal rigidity: Head flexion resulting from spasm of posterior neck muscles
- Kernig's sign: In supine, flex thigh and fully to chest, then extend knee; causes spasm of Hamstrings, resistance, and pain

- Brudzinski's sign: In supine, flex head to chest causes flexion of both legs (drawing up)
- Irritability: Restlessness, disorientation, photophobia
- General weakness
- Neck movements
- SLR (Straight Leg Raising test)
- Meningeal irritation.

## ASSESS MOTOR SYSTEM

### Strength Scales

- Medical Research Council (MRC) scale (grade 0-5) (Table 1.1)
- Manual Muscle test (MMT) (Table 1.2)
- Clinically to evaluate muscle strength adequately without resorting to special equipment:
  - Dynamometers
  - Myometers
  - Ergometer

| Table 1.1: The Medical Research counil scale of muscle strength ( Mendell and Florence, 1990). Figs 1.5 and 1.6 |
|---|
| 0 No contraction |
| 1 A flicker or trace of contraction |
| 2 Active movement with gravity eliminated |
| 3 Active movement against gravity |
| 4 Active movement against gravity and moderate resistance |
| 5 Normal Power. |

- The muscle strength scale by physical therapist's grades muscle on a six-point scale from zero (no motion) through trace, poor, fair and good to normal.

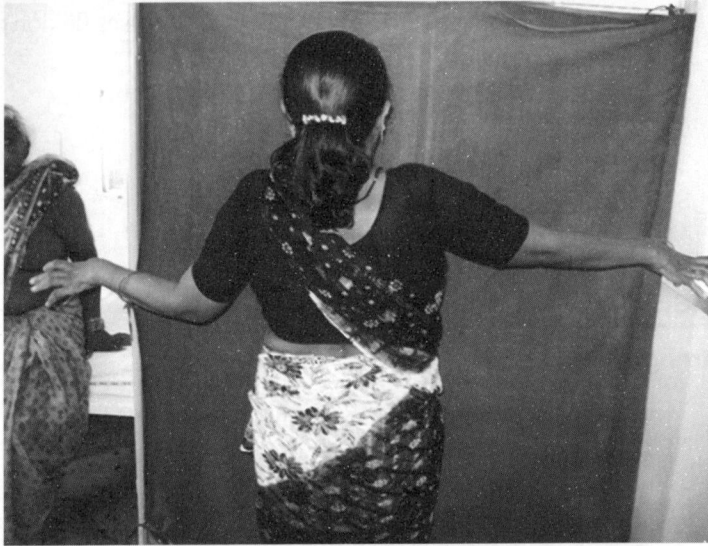

Fig. 1.5: Bilateral abductor muscle weakness

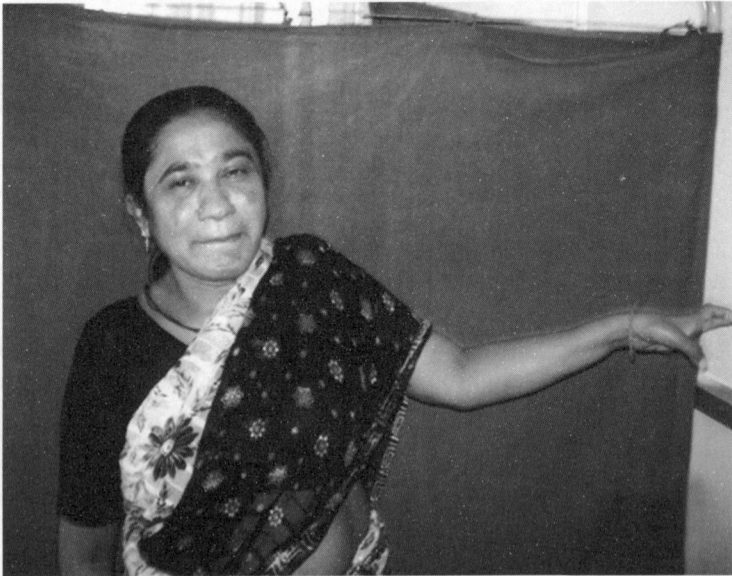

Fig. 1.6: Difficult to raise left shoulder (abductor muscle weakness)

| Table 1.2 : Segmentation and Innervations of the muscles to joints ||
|---|---|
| **Upper extremity** ||
| Abduction of shoulders | C5 |
| Adduction of shoulder | C5 |
| Flexion of shoulder | C5 |
| Extension of elbow | C7 |
| Flexion of wrist | C6, 7, 8 |
| Extension of wrist | C6, 7 |
| Finger movements | C8, T1 |
| **Lower extremity** ||
| Flexion of hip | L1, 2, 3 |
| Extension of hip | L5, S1 |
| Adduction of hip | L5, S1 |
| Flexion of knee | L4, 5, S1, 2 |
| Extension of knee | L3, 4 |
| Dorsiflexion of foot | L4, 5 |
| Plantar flexion | S1 |
| Inversion of foot | L4 |
| Eversion of foot | L5, 6 |
| Dorsiflexion of toes | L5 |

## ASSESS MUSCLE TONE

- Tone is difficult to assess. The examination of tone requires a relaxed muscles.

### Methods

- Inspection
- Muscle palpation
- Passive manipulation—to assess the extensibility, flexibility and range of motion
- The limb is moved passively, first slowly and through a complete range of motion, and then at varying speeds.

*Neurological Examination*

## Abnormalities of Tone (Hypotonia) (Fig. 1.7)

*Example*

- Cerebellar Disease
- Chorea
- Infantile Hypotonia (Floppy Baby syndrome)
- Hemiparesis.

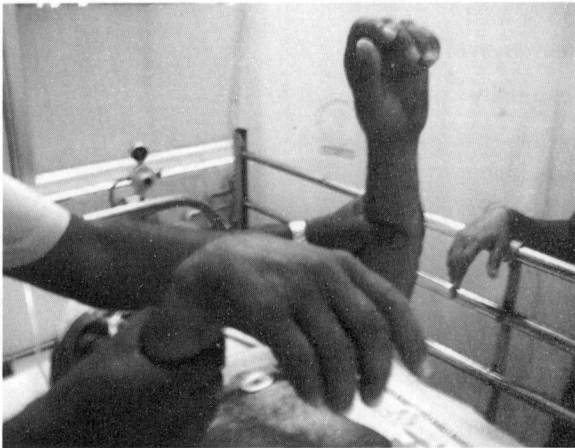

**Fig. 1.7:** Test muscle tone: Flaccid paralysis/No response, usually complete flexed at the right wrist (Hand drops). Left wrist is in normal position.

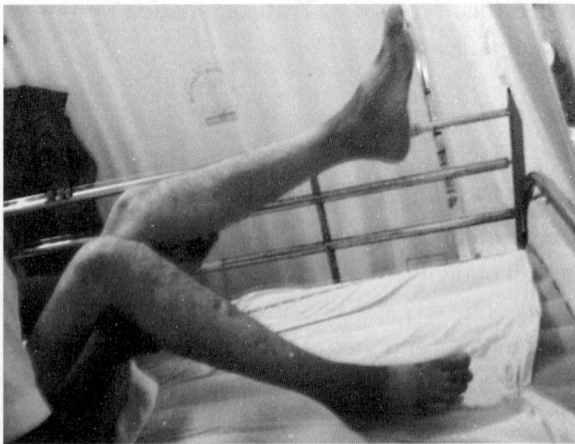

**Fig. 1.8:** Right knee in complete flexed pattern/left lower limb is normal.

## Hypertonia (Fig. 1.8)

*Example*

- Extrapyramidal Rigidity
- Spasticity
- Epilepsy, seizures, tetany.

## ASSESS MUSCLE VOLUME AND CONTOUR

### Examination

- Inspection
- Palpation
- Measurement ( Tape Measure or Calipers)
- Muscle atrophy (Amyotrophy) - Decrease in muscle volume or Bulk.
    - Changes in shape or contour.
- Muscle Hyper trophy - An increase in the bulk or volume of muscle tissues.

### Abnormalities of Volume and Contour

*Indications*

- Muscle atrophy (Figs.1.9 and 1.10)
    - E. g. : Diseases of anterior horn cells, root or peripheral nerve
    - Congential Hemiplegia
    - Myogenic atrophy

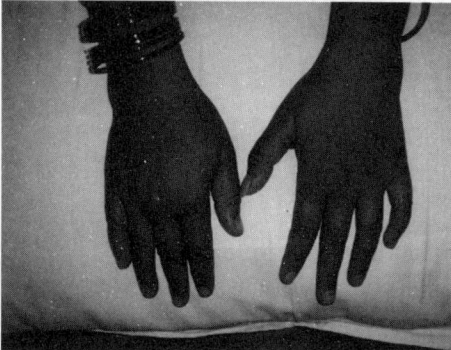

**Fig. 1.9:** Disuse atrophy of the left intrinsic muscles of little finger/Right side little finger is normal

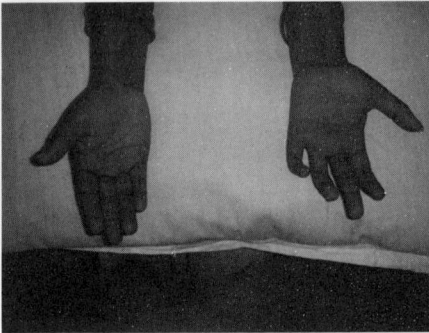

**Fig. 1.10:** Disuse atrophy of the left intrinsic muscles of little finger/hight side little finger is normal

- Neurogenic atrophy:
    - E.g.: Bell's palsy or peripheral nerve injury
    - Amyotrophic lateral sclerosis
    - Progressive spinal muscular atrophy
    - Peroneal muscular atrophy
    - Muscular dystrophy, pseudo hypertrophy.

### Assess Abnormalities of Movement

- Assess the abnormal, involuntary, unwanted movements (Hyperkinetic movement disorders).

*Example*

- Parkinson's Disease (Abnormally decreased movement)
- Chorea
- Hemiballismus
- Dystonia (to abnormally increased movement)
- Tremor
- Myoclonus
- Fasciculations
- Spasms.

### Assess Reflexes (Table 1.3)

- Erb introduced the term tendon reflex in 1875
- Reflex is an involuntary response to a sensory stimulus
- Reflexes elicited by application of a stretch stimulus to either tendons or periosteum or occasionally to bones, joints, fascia or

aponeurotic structures are usually referred to as muscle stretch or deep tendon reflexes
- Best tested using a high quality Rubber Percussion Hammer or Taylor (Tomahawk) Hammer
- Reflexes are reduced or absent in lower motor neurone and brisk or exaggerated in upper motor neurone lesion.

| Table 1.3 : The Common Deep Tendon (Muscle stretch) Reflexes (Figs 1.11 A to D) | | |
|---|---|---|
| Reflex | Segmental Level | Peripheral Nerve |
| Biceps | C5-6 | Musculocutaneous |
| Triceps | C7- 8 | Radial |
| Brachioradialis | C5-6 | Radial |
| Quadriceps | L3-4 | Femoral |
| Achilles | S1 | Sciatic |

*Reflex Score*

0  Absent
1  Decreased reflex
2  Normal response
3  Exaggerated
4  Hyperactive

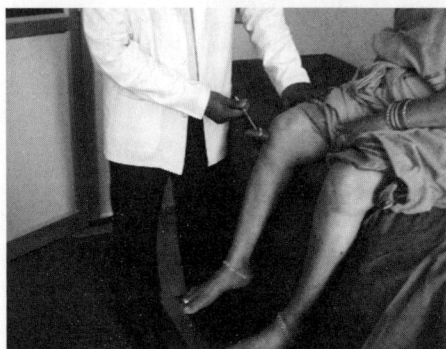

**Fig. 1.11A:** Knee jerk

**Assess Superficial Reflexes**

- May be indicated for central nervous system and peripheral nervous system lesions (e.g. : Spinal cord injury, stroke)

Neurological Examination

Neurological Examination

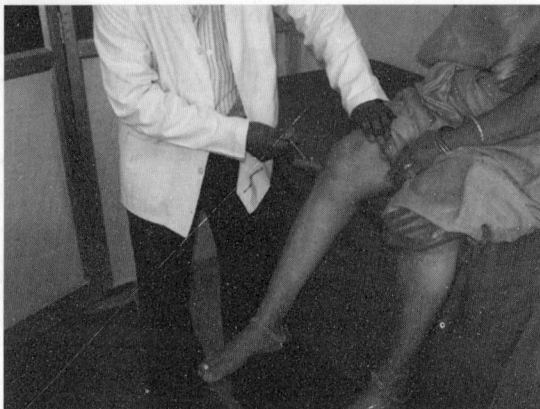

**Fig. 1.11.B:**
Knee jerk

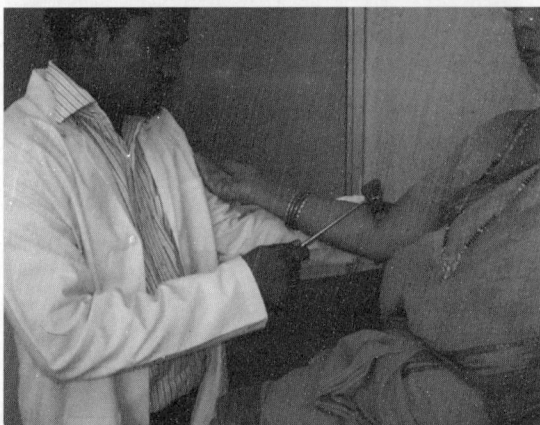

**Fig. 1.11C:**
Biceps jerk

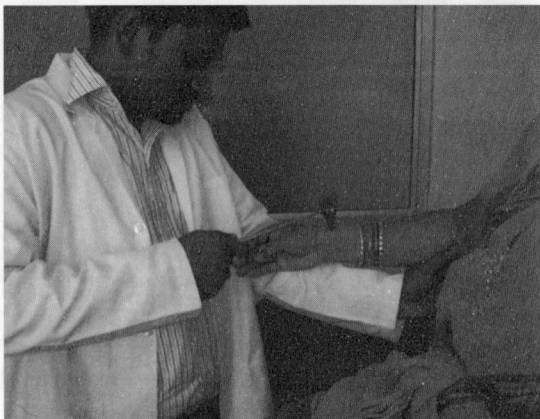

**Fig. 1. 11D:**
Supinator jerk

- Abdominal reflex: A light stroke applied over of the four quadrants of the abdomen will, in the normal individual, elicit a brisk contraction of the understanding muscles
- The upper reflexes segments T9- T10
- The Lower reflexes segments T11- T12
- The symmetry of the abdominal reflex response, since its absence on one side may be good evidence of an upper motor neuron lesion.

## Plantar Response

- Applying a firm pressure along the lateral border of the dorsum of the foot and observing the metarsophalangeal joint of the great toe
- In normal circumstance the toe flexors (goes down)
- In pyramidal and corticospinal lesions (upper motor neurone) the great toe shows an extensor response (it goes up, with an associated fanning of the toes)
- Babinski sign: Great toe extension (S1-2) Figs. 1.12 and 1.13
- Positive Babinski is an abnormal response to plantar reflex testing.

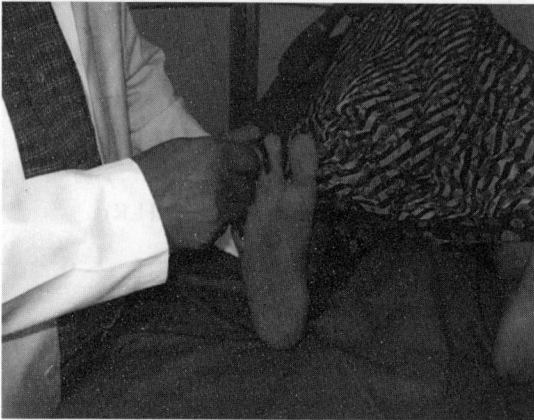

**Fig. 1.12:** Babinski response

## Assess Primitive and Spinal Reflexes

- Tonic/Brainstem reflexes may be indicated in CNS lesions (stroke, traumatic brain injury).

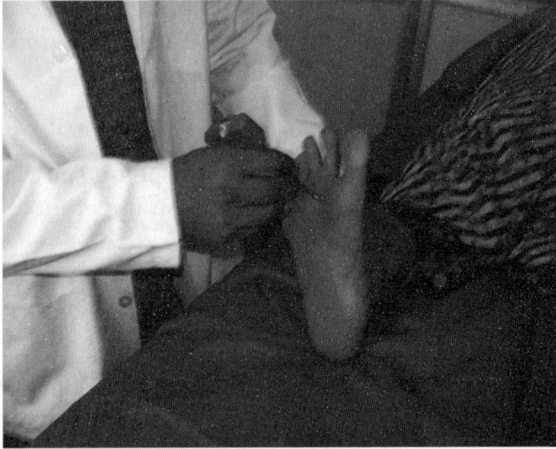

**Fig. 1.13:** Babinski response

## Reflexes Tested

*Primitive/Spinal*

- Flexor withdrawal
- Crossed extension
- Traction
- Grasp.

*Tonic/Brain Stem*

- Asymmetrical tonic neck reflex (ATNR)
- Symmetrical tonic neck reflex (STNR)
- Symmetrical tonic labyrinthine reflex (STLR)
- Positive support, associated reactions.

*Score*

**Scale range from**

  0 absent
  1 Tone change; no visible movement of extremities
  2+ Visible movement of extremities
  3+ Exaggerated, full movement of extremities
  4+ Obligatory and sustained movement, lasting for more than 30
    seconds.

Neurological Examination

## Assess Midbrain/ Cortical Reactions

- Righting reactions
- Protective reactions
- Equilibrium reactions.

## Sensory System Assessment

- To assess superficial sensations ask patient to describe where sensation does not feel normal; provided sensory clues.

*Five basic modalities of Sensation*

1. Pain
2. Temperature
3. Light touch
4. Vibration sense
5. Joint position sense.
- Pain: Test sharp/dull sensation in response to sharp/dull stimuli with disposable safety pin or paper clip
- Temperature: Test hot/ cold sensation in response to hot/cold stimuli tubes filled with hot/cold
- Touch: Test touch/not touch in response to slight touch stimulus (Cotton ball or no touch).

## Assess Proprioceptive Sensations (Table 1.4)

- Joint Position Sense: Ask the patient to closure his/her eyes; more the patient's limb (Up or down/ in or out)
- Vibration Sense: Test Propriceptive pathways by applying vibrating fork the bony prominences
- Movement Sense (Kinesthesia): Test ability to perceive movement in response to your moving the patient's limb. Patient can duplicate movement with opposite limb or give a verbal report.

| Table 1.4: The Sensory (Dermatome) Innervations |
| --- |
| • C2 - Occipital |
| • C3 - Lateral Cervical area |
| • C4 - Tip of Scapula |
| • C5 - Lateral aspect of elbow |
| • C6 - Thumb |
| • C7 - Middle finger |

*Neurological Examination*

*Contd...*

*Contd...*

- C8 - Little finger
- T1 - Inner aspect of elbow
- T3 - Axilla
- T8 - Costal region
- T10 - Umbilicus
- T12 - Pubis
- L1 - Below Inguinal ligament
- L3 - Knee
- L4 - Medial surface of tibia
- L5 - Outer aspect of tibia to inner aspect of foot and great toe
- S1 - Lateral aspect of foot and little toe.

## ASSESS CORTICAL SENSATIONS

### Stereognosis

- The perception, understanding and identification of the form and nature of objects by touch.

### Graphesthesia

- The ability to recognize letters or numbers written on the skin, with a pencil, dull pain or similar object
- Normal response is correctly identifying the written letter or number.

### Two-Point Discrimination

- Test by placing two points of stimulus on the patients skin and gradually bringing them together until there is one-point stimulus
- The patient is asked to determine if there is one point or two points and when they come together to one point.

### Barognosis

- Test by placing an object in the patient's hand and requesting the patient to respond if it is heavier or lighter than the previous object.

### Texture

- Test by placing different textures sample cotton, wool, silk or leather in the patients hand and asking the patient to identify the texture.

## Kinesthesia

- Moving the patient's extremity up, down, out or in. The patient is asked to describe the movement by the therapist.

## TESTING OF COORDINATION

### Finger to Nose Test

- The patient extends the arm completely and then touches the tip of the index finger to the tip of the nose, slowly at first, then rapidly, with the eyes open and then closed
- If the patient is not fluent, then you should ask him/her to repeat the action of touching his/her nose with the eyes closed
- Example: Cerebellar disease.

### Heel-to-Shin Test

- To assess lower limb coordination
- Ask the patient to slide the heel of one foot in a straight line down the shin of the other leg
- In cerebellar ataxia, the heel wavers across the intended target.

### Dysdiadochokinesia

- Dysdiadochokinesia is an inability to perform rapidly repeated movements
- Test: Ask the patient to pretend to screw a light bulb into a socket
- Another test is to ask the patient to perform simple repetitive movements, such as drawing a circle with a finger on the back of one and then the other
- Slow, awkward movements indicate dysdiadochokinesia.

### Romberg's Test

- A simple test to determine whether an ataxic gait (a patients's unsteadiness) results form a cerebellar or proprioception lesion
- The patient is asked to stand with feet together and then to close his/her eyes
- Where there is loss of proprioception, the patient immediately loses stability (Positive Romberg's Test).

## GAIT ASSESSMENT

## Methods

- Observation
- Gait analysis and Motion Lab
- EMG Biofeedback
- Assess length of step, width of base
- Abnormal leg movements
- Instability
- Associated postural movements.

## BIBLIOGRAPHY

- Adams RD, Victor M. Prinicples of Neurology, New york: Mc-Graw Hill, 2008.
- Brain Wr. Diseases of the nervous system; Oxford University press, London, 1933; p. 899.
- Ballinger A, Patchett S. Clinical medicine, China, 3rd: Saunders, Elsevier, 2005; p. 635-720.
- Carr JH, Shepherd RB. Physiotherapy Disorders of the Brain. London, Heineman, 1990.
- Donagly M, Neurology. Oxford Press, 2004.
- Fuller G. Neurological Examination Made easy. Edinburg: Churchill Livingstone, 2006.
- Gajdosik RL, Bohannon RW. Clinical Measurement of Range of motion: review of goinometry emphasizing reliability and validity. Physical Therapy, 1987; 67: 1867-72.
- Harms Ringdahl K. Muscle Strength. Edinburg: Churchill Livingstone, 1993.
- Lincoln N, Leadbitter D. Assessment of Motor function in Stroke patients, Physiotherapy, 1979; 65; 48-51.
- Lance TW. What is Spasticity? Lancet, 1990; 335- 606.
- Loewen SC, Anderson BA. Reliability of the modified motor Assessment scale and the Barthel Index. Physiotherapy, 1988; 68: 1077-81.
- Mahoney FL, Barthel BW. Functional Evaluation; The Barthel Index. Maryland Stroke Med J, 1965; 14; 61-5.
- Teasdale G, Murray G, Parker L, et. al. Adding up the Glasgow Coma Scale, Acta Neurosurgical, suppl, 1979;28;13-6.
- Van Gijn J - The Babinski sign and the pyramidal syndrome, J. Neurol, Neuro surg, Psychiaat, 1978; 41;865-73.
- Wade DT - Measurement in Neurological Rehabilitation. Current Opinion in Neurology, 1993; 6: 778-84.

Neurological Examination

*Chapter*

*//////////////////////////////*

# ② 

# Neuroradiology Imaging

**Neuroradiology Imaging**

## PLAIN RADIOGRAPHY: SKULL X-RAY

- Conversion of motion energy into radiant energy produces X-ray
- Radiography of the skull is carried out with reference to visible or palpable landmarks and recognized lines and planes of the skull
- In neurological referral, the recommended projections are:
  - Lateral
  - Occipitofrontal
  - Frontoocciptal
  - Submento vertical
- Immobilization of the patient is essential if high quality radiograph of skull are to be produced
- Aids in imaging integrity of bone table, identifying lesions of bone, corresponding with pain or cranial nerve dysfunction (Wilhelm conrad Roentgen 1895).

## COMPUTER TOMOGRAPHY (CT SCAN)

- Computed tomography (GN Hounsfield 1970)— It is a noninvasive neuroimaging technique
- CT scan provides a means of producing transverse axial tomographic images of a patient
- Plays vital role in accident and emergency cases where its ability to produce high quality images with minimal disturbance to patient is particularly valuable
- Modality of choice for imaging acute head trauma— Hemorrhages, contusions, Facial- Clavicle fractures
- In identifying calcified primary brain tumors, extra axial tumors in adults, metastasis
- Best evaluation in fractures of spine
- In axial back pain, injection of contrast materials into nucleus of intervertebral disc followed by CT Discography
- Use to imaging osseous structures of the spine, skull base and temporal bones (William PD, 2001).

## MAGNETIC RESONANCE IMAGING (MRI SCAN, DAMADIAN, 1977)

- MRI is an application of the principle of hydrogen atoms in the patient's tissue is examined
- While scan times are longer, soft tissue differentiation is excellent and often possible to distinguish abnormal from normal tissue
- Provides best and most direct evaluations of contents with in spinal cord along with interverebral discs, ligaments, musculature and aids in detection of degenerative disorders (Cervical, Thoracic, Lumbao-sacral spine) (Richard TK, et.al 2009)
- Contraindications: Metal implants, Pacemakers.

### Myelography

- Radiography of spine following injection of an opaque substance into the lumbar spinal subarachnoid space, usually at the L2- L3
- For diagnosis of diseases of the spinal cord and canal (e.g. Syringomyelia, Paraplegia
- Evaluation of suspected meningeal or arachnoid cysts and the localization of spinal dural arterio venous fistulas and CSF fistulas
- Contraindications: Post Headache, vomiting and meningitis.

### Ventriculography

- X-ray of skull following injection of air into lateral ventricles
- Useful with to increased intracranial pressures.

### Angiography

- Evaluation of patients with vascular pathology
- Indication: For patients intra cranial small vessel pathology (such as vasculitis) aneurysms, and vascular malformations
- Complications: atherosclerosis, vasospasm, low Cardiac output and subarachnoid hemorrhage.

## POSITION EMISSION TOMOGRAPHY (PET)

- PET in which radioisotopes are inhaled or injected and emissions are measured with a gamma ray detector system
- A major clinical tool for imaging cerebral blood flow and brain metabolism.

### Neuromuscular Diagnostic Tests

*Electroencephalography (Berger, 1929)*

- Is the method of recording changes of potential in the brain
- Recording of electrical activity of brain, appearing as periodic waves
- The principal use of EEG is in the diagnosis of epilepsy and seizures (Hill. D. 1995).

*Electromyography (EMG)*

- EMG the recording of electrical changes present in muscles at rest or evoked by voluntary movement
- The record is made by introducing a concentric needle into the muscle to be tested
- When a normal muscle is completely relaxed, no electrical activity can be detected in it.

*Indication*

- Lesions of the lower motor neuron
- Myotonia, myasthenia gravis
- Measure recovery after a peripheral nerve lesion
- It is useful in the diagnosis of neuromuscular diseases such as motor neuron disease, muscular dystrophy and poliomyelitis.

### Nerve Conduction Velocity (NCV)

- Nerve conduction velocity along the sensory or motor component of a peripheral nerve can be measured by recording the sensory or motor response from a site of electrical stimulation
- This technique is used in the diagnosis of entrapment syndrome,

carpel tunnel syndrome, compression of median nerve and diagnosis of peripheral neuropathy (axonal or demyelization).

## Evoked Potentials

- External, auditory or somatosensory stimuli are used to evoke potentials in brain
- Visual evoked potential (VEP)
- Brain auditory evoked potential (BAEP)
- Somato sensory evoked potential (SEP)
- Potentials are recorded by from surface electrodes and processed by computer
- Delineates conduction times along there sensory pathways
- Detects lesions if responses are delayed or absent.

## Lumbar Puncture (LP)

- A Lumbar puncture insertion of spinal needle below level of L1-L2
- Examination of CSF, particularly in patients of meningitis, subarachnoid hemorrhage and suspected inflammatory brain disease (Thomspson 1995)
- Measures intra cranial pressures and spinal fluid dynamics
- Complications: infection, epidural hematoma, herination.

## Muscle Biopsy

- The Chief use is to detect inflammatory myopathies particularly in inflammatory disorders such as polymyositis, degenerative disorders such as the muscular dystrophies (Dubowitz and Brooke 1973)
- Help to identify a neurogenic atrophy by the uniformity of enzyme activity in the reinnervated fibers
- The biopsy is taken from an affected muscle and then processed for light and electron microscopy
- Use to identify the different muscle fiber types and abnormalities in specific enzyme pathways.

## BIBLIOGRAPHY

- Adams RD, et al. Prinicples of Neurology. 5th ed, Newyork; Mc Graw-Hill, 1997.
- David O. Wiebers, et al. Mayo Clinic Examinations in Neurology. 7th ed, Mosby, 1998; p. 331- 511.
- Dillon WP. Neuroimaging in Neurologic Disorders, Mc Graw-Hill, New York, 2001; p. 2337-41.
- Donaghy. M. Brain's Diseases of the Nervous System. 11th ed, Oxford University press, 2001.
- Fuller G. Neurological Examination made easy. Newyork; Churchill Livingstone, 1999.
- Frackowiak, RSJ. Positron emission tomography in neurology. In Recent advances in Clinical neurology. vol. 5; Edinburgh, Churchill Livingstone, 1988; p. 239-77.
- Gilliatt. RW. Clinical Electromyography in Modern trends in Neurology, Willams, London, 1957; p. 65.
- Hill.D. Encephalography in Recent Advances in Neurology and Psychiatry, ed Brain WR and Strauss EB, 6th ed, London, 1995; 113-14.
- Kimura J. Electro Diagnosis in Diseases of Nerve and Muscle, 2nd ed, Philadelphia, Davis, 1989.
- Susan B.O' Sullivan. Neurological Physical Therapy. APTA; International Educational Resource Ltd, Massachusetts, USA, 2006.
- Scott, WA. Magnetic Resonance Imaging of the Brain and Spine. 4th ed, Lippincott willams and Wilkins, 2009.
- Sir Roger Bannister. Brain and Bannister's Clincal Neurology, 7th ed; Oxford University press; 2004; p. 211- 36.
- Warlow, C. Hand Book of Neurology. Oxford, Blackwell scientific Publications, 1991.

Neuroradiology Imaging

# Chapter

## 3

# Physical Therapy in Bell's Palsy

## BELL'S PALSY

Sir Charles Bell (1821) described the Facial (Bell's) Palsy. It is a complex neuromuscular facial disorder or unknown etiology commonly affecting the motor neurons of facial muscles receiving their neurological innervations from the seventh cranial nerve (Vanswearinggen and Brach 1998).

### Etiology

- Cold exposure is a frequent cause, for example driving with a car window open in frigid weather or sleeping with window open a chilly night
- Inflammation and edema
- Herpes Zoster Virus (HZV)
- Facial Trauma (e.g. Obstetric forceps)
- Ramsay Hunt syndrome
- Postacoustic neuromas surgery
- Some cases have recently being reported after inflammation of intranasal influenza vaccine.

### Incidence

The incidence of Bell's palsy is also higher in patients with diabetes as compared to the general population. It affects both sexes equally and is less frequent in children than adults.

### Clinical Manifestations (Figs. 3.1 to 3.5)

- Idiopathic facial (Bell's) palsy is the most common conditions seen in neurologic practice
- Pain behind the ipsilateral ear in the mastoid region for a day or two before the onset of weakness
- Facial paralysis is often maximal at onset or may progress for over 24 to 48 hours
- Eye brow droops and cannot be elevated
- Impaired drainage of the tears, which overflow on to the cheek
- Problems with eating and drinking and transient disturbance or oropharyngeal swallowing is approximately 2/3rd of patients

- Angle of the mouth droops
- Loss of taste sensation or hyperacusis (an unpleasant quality to louder sounds)
- Dryness of the eye or mouth
- Twitching.

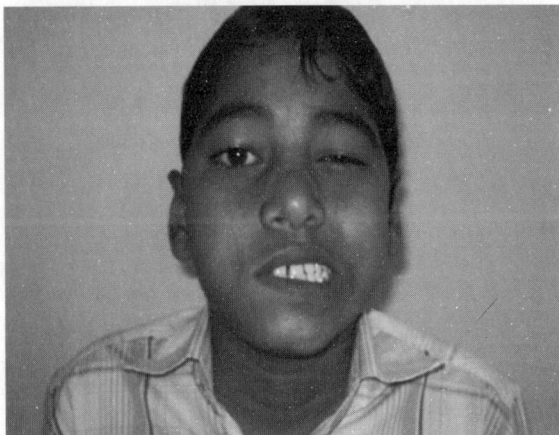

**Fig. 3.1:** Mouth deviation

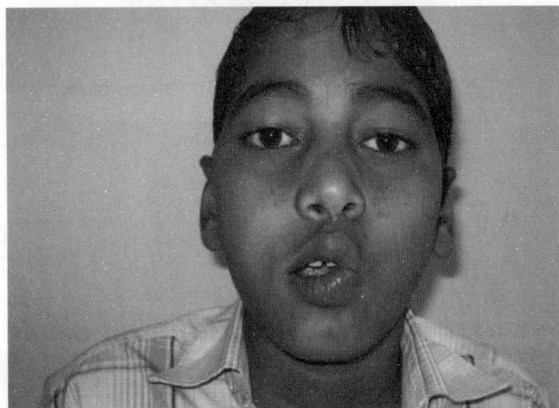

**Fig. 3.2:** Weakness of the right orbicularis oris muscle

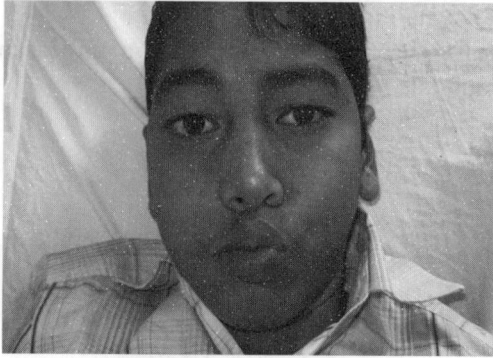

**Fig. 3.3:** Mentalis muscle weakness

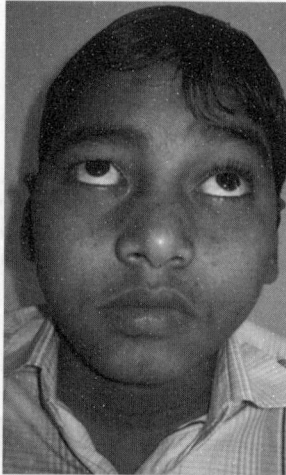

**Fig. 3.4:** Difficulty to raise right forehead muscle

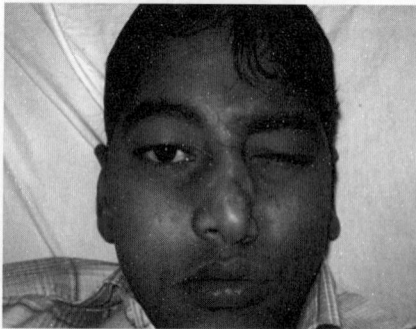

**Fig. 3.5:** Nasalis muscle weakness

Physical Therapy in Bell's Palsy

## Diagnosis

*EMG Test*

- The severity and the extent of nerve involvement and the presence of nerve damage is determined.

*X-Ray*

- Can help rule out infection or tumor.

*MRI/ CT scan*

- Can eliminate other causes of pressure on the facial nerve.

## Special Tests

- Facial nerve grading system (House JW, Brackmann DE,1985) (Table 3.1)

## Assessment

- Observe for drooping of mouth, eyelid's that don't close
- Assess function of facial muscle expression (wrinkle forehead, raised eyebrows, frown, smile, close eyes, tightly puff checks)
- Assess taste of the anterior 2/3rd of tongue.

| Table: 3.1: House -Brackmann Facial Narve Scale, 1985 | | |
|---|---|---|
| Grade | Description | Findings |
| I | Normal | Normal facial function in all areas. |
| II | Mild dysfunction | Gross: Sight weakness on close inspection, very slight synkiesis.<br>At rest: Normal symmetry and tone.<br>In motion: Forhead - moderate to good function<br>Eye – complete closure with minimal effort<br>Mouth – slight aysmmetric. |

*Contd...*

Contd...

| Grade | Description | Findings |
|-------|-------------|----------|
| III | Moderate dysfunction | Gross: Obvious but not disfiguring difference between sides; Noticeable but not severe synkinesis. At rest: Normal symmetry and tone. In motion: Forehead – slight to moderate movement; Eye – complete closure with effort; Mouth - slightly week with maximal effort. |
| IV | Moderate severe dysfunction | Gross: Obvious weakness or disfiguring asymmetry. At rest: Normal symmetry and tone. In motion: Forhead – no movement; eye– incomplete closure; Mouth – slight movement. |
| V | Total Paralysis | No movement. |

## PHYSICAL THERAPY INTERVENTION

### Aims

- To educate/reassure the patient about the condition
- Reestabilizing facial movements and strength (Marcia RA, et.al 2007)
- To relief pain
- To reeducate sensation if involved sensory integration (touch, two point discrimination, temperature)
- To improve muscle contraction
- To prevent complications.

Physical therapy management to achieve the mentioned goals are as follows: Electro thermo therapy, facial manipulation, sensory stimulation, Kobat technique and guidence, stretching, Facial active ROM exercise, Neuromuscular training, High voltage therapy, EMG biofeedback.

### Patient Education

- Explain the condition to the patient; its cause, incidence, prognosis and treatment

Physical Therapy in Bell's Palsy

- Explain to the patient that following the Physical therapy program is enough
- Don't expose yourself to direct sunlight, being too close to TV light or strong room lighting
- Wear sun glasses to protect eyes
- Do not exhaust eyes by reading for long time
- Avoid direct contact with air conditioners.

## Electrothermo Therapy

### Electrical Stimulation (ES)

- ES of paralyzed muscles has long been a popular intervention for patients with Bell's palsy
- Six facial muscles (Frontalis, Orbularis oculi, Oribularis oris, Zygomaticus major, Nasalis and Triangularis)
- Pulsed electrical stimulation to reduce neuromuscular conduction latencies and minimize clinical impairments in patients with by standing facial nerve damage (Farragher, et al)
- To improve motor recovery in patients with acute and chronic Bell's palsy (Patrica JO and Michelle Lz, et al. 2006).

### Ultrasound

- Ultrasound can be beneficial for acute Bell's palsy
- To reduce edema and provide normal healing environment.

### EMG Biofeedback

- EMG Biofeedback is more effective and significantly improved symmetry of voluntary movement and linear measurement of facial expression (Ross. et al. 1991).

### Pulsed Short wave Diathermy (PSWD)

- Pulsed short wave diathermy can facilitate healing process in acute condition
- No evidence supports the benefit of using continues mode of short wave diathermy.

*Laser*

- Laser, still has no study supporting to use it with acute or chronic condition.

## Neuromuscular Retraining (NMT)

- Neuromuscular retraining (NMT) is applied using selective motor training to facilitate symmetrical movement and control undesired gross motor activity
- Patient reeducation is the most important aspect of the treatment process
- EMG biofeedback and or a specific exercise will provide a sensory feedback to promote learning
- When each muscle group is being assessed, the patient observes action of these muscles in the mirror and instructed to perform small symmetrical specific movements on sound side to identify the right response
- Patient can begin to perform exercise to improve facial movements guided by affected side so isolated muscle response is preserved and coordination improved
- Repetitions and frequency of exercise can be modified according to improvement status
- The movements should be initiated slowly and gradually so that the patient can observe the angle, strength and speed of each movement, because rapid movements can't help the patient in controlling the abnormal movement (synkinesis).

## Stretching

- Stretching is recommended here to prevent muscle tightness.

## Facial Manipulation

- Facial manipulation can be performed in conjunction with other treatment options. It can be done to improve perceptual awareness
- Facial manipulations on the face include:
  - Effleurage
  - Finger or thumb kneading
  - Wringing
  - Hacking
  - Tapping
  - Stroking.

## Kabat Rehabilitation

- Kabat techniques are a type of motor control rehabilitation technique based on Proprioceptive neuromuscular facilitation (PNF)
- During Kabat, therapist facilitate the voluntary contraction of the impaired muscle by applying a global stretching then resistance to the entire muscular section and the motivate action by verbal input and manual contact
- Prior to Kabat, ice stimulation has to perform a specific muscular group in order to increase its contractile power (Barbara et al. 2010).

## BIBLIOGRAPHY

- Adour KK, Ruboyianes JM, Trent CS, et al. Bell's Palsy treatment with acyclovir and prednisone with compared with prednisone alone: A double blind, randomized controlled trial; Ann Oto Rhin and Largng vol:105; Issue, 1999;5:371-8.
- Brach JS, Vanswearingen JM. Not all facial paralysis is Bell's palsy: A Case report. Arch Phys Med Rehab, 1999;80:857-9.
- Buttress S, Herren K. Electrical stimulation and Bell's palsy (Best evidence Topic Report). Emerg Med J; 2002;19: 428.
- Barbara, Maurizo, et al. Role of Kabat Physical rehabilitation in Bell's palsy, Acta Oto Laryngoloica, No: 1, March , 2010; 130: 167-72 (6).
- Cronin GW, Steenerson RL. The Effectiveness of Neuromuscular facial retraining combined with electromyography in facial paralysis Rehabilitation. Otolaryngology. Head and Neck surgery, 2003;128: p 534-8.
- Centre for Reviews and Dissemination: The efficacy of electrotherapy for Bell's Palsy: A systemic review (Provisional Record). Database of abstracts of Reviews of effectiveness, 2005; issue: 4.
- Diels HJ. Facial Paralysis: is there a role for a Therapist. Facial Plast surg, 2000;16: p 361-4.
- Dalla T, Elena, Bossi, Daniela, et al. Usefulness of BFB/EMG in facial Palsy Rehabilitation. Disab and Rehab, 2005; Vol:27, No: 14: p. 809-15.
- Elisabet CW, Monika FO, Per H, Ingemer F. Evaluation of a Physiotherapeutic treatment intervention in Bell's Palsy. Physio Ther Pract, 2006; vol 22 (no:1): p. 43-52.
- Farragher D, Kidd GL, Tallis R. Eutrophic Electrical stimulation for Bell's palsy. Clinical Rehabilitation; 1987;1:265-71.
- Fernado CK, Basmajian JV. Biofeedback in Physical medicine and rehabilitation, Biofeedback and self Regulation. Task Force Report of BSA; 1978; vol 3 (no: 4).

- Frach JP, Osterbaner PJ, Fuhr AW. Treatment of Bell's Palsy by mechanical force, manually assisted chiropractic adjusting and High voltage electrotherapy. J Manipulative Physio Ther; 1992;15; 596-98.
- Gahimer JE, Domholdt E. Amount of patient education in Physical therapy practice and Perceived effects. Phys Ther, 1996;76:1089- 96.
- Holland NJ, Weiner GM. Recent Development in Bell's Palsy, BMJ, 2004; 329: 553-7.
- House JW, Brackmann DE. Facial Nerve Grading system, Otolaryngol Head Neck Surg, 1985;93;146-7.
- Jennifer SB, Jessie M, Vanswearingen. Case Reports-Physical therapy for facial paralysis: A tailored approach. Phys Ther, 1999; vol 79 ( no: 4) (Aprl 1): 397-404.
- Lindsay RW, Robinson M, Hadlock.TA. Comprehensive Facial Rehabilitation improves function in people with facial Parlaysis: A 5 year experience at the Massachusetts eye and Ear Infirmary. Phy Ther; Mar 1, 2010; 90(3): 371-78.
- Mosforth J, Taverner D. Physiotherapy for Bell's palsy. BMJ 1958;2: 675-7.
- Margaret Hollis. Massage for Therapists. Blackwell scientific publications, oxford, 1992 .
- Marcia RG, Jefferson RC, Alessandrade mG, et al. Physical Therapy on Peripheral facial paralysis: Retrospective study. Braziijan J Otorhinololarynology, 1999;73 (1): 112-5.
- Manikandan. Effect of Facial neuromuscular reeducation on facial symmetry in patients with Bell's palsy: A randomized controlled trial, Clin Rehab; Apr 1, 2007; 90(3): 391-397.
- Nakamura K, Toda N, et.al. Biofeedback Rehabilitation for prevention of synkinesis after facial palsy, Otolaryngol Head Neck Surg, 2003' 128: 539-43.
- On AY, Yaltirik HP, Kirazli.Y. Agreement between clinical and Electromyographic assessment during the course of peripheral facial paralysis. Clin Rehab; April 1, 2007; 21(4): 344-50.
- Peiterson E. Natural History of Bell's Palsy, AmJ Otol 1982;4:107-11.
- Quinn R, Cramp F. The efficacy of electrotherapy for Bell's palsy: A systemic review, Phys Ther Reviews 2003;8:151-64.
- Spielholz NI. Electrical stimulation of dennervated muscle In Nelson RM, Hayes KW, Currier DP. eds: Clinical Electrotherapy, 3rd Ed, Stanford, Appleton and Lange: 1999; Chapter 9.
- Shrode LW. Treatment of facial muscles affected by Bell's palsy by mechanical force, manually assisted chiropractic adjusting and High voltage electrotherapy. J Manipulative Physio Ther; 1992;15:596-98.
- Targan RS, Alon G, and Kay SL. Effect of long-term Electrical stimulation on motor recovery and improvement of clinical residuals in patients with unresolved facial nerve palsy, Otolaryngol Head neck surgery 2000; P. 246-52.
- William, Bierman. Diagnosis and Treatment of Bell's palsy, JAMA, vol: 149: no: May 17, 1952;3.

# Chapter

## 4

# Stroke Physical Therapy

## STROKE

The term of Stroke (or) Cerbrovascular Accident (CVA) is a sudden focal neurologic deficit resulting from ischemic or hemorrhagic lesion in the brain (O'sullivan 2004). Approximately 80% of strokes are caused by to little blood flow (ischemic stroke) and the remaining 20% are nearly equally between hemorrhage into brain tissue (parenchymatous hemorrhage) and hemorrage into the surrounding subarchnoid space (Subarachnoid Hemorrhage).

## CEREBROVASCULAR ANATOMY

Most of strokes caused by abnormalities with in the cerebral circulation, an understanding of cerebraovascular anatomy helps in arriving at the correct diagnosis and determining the underlying pathogenesis and prognosis.

The brain is supplied by four major arteries:
1. The left and right internal carotid artery and vertebral arteries.
2. The left common carotid artery aries from aortic arch, but the other vessels originate from branches of the aorta.
3. The right common carotid artery.
4. The left and right vertebral arteries.

### Epidemiology

- Third leading cause of death (1 of every 14.5 deaths after heart disease and cancer in world wide)
- 72% of strokes occur in patients occur in patients > 65 years of age
- 14% of patients have a transient ischemic attack (TIA) within one year
- 50-70% of stroke survivors regain functional independence, whereas 15-30% are permanently disabled (Brammer CM, et al 2002).

### Classification

- Transient Ischemic Attack (TIA): An acute loss of focal cerebral or monocular function with symptoms lasting less than 24 hours which after adequate investigation, is presumed to be due to embolus or thrombotic vascular disease (War low and Morris 1982)

- Ischemic Stroke: Results from interference with blood circulation to the brain (Table 4.1). The precise signs and symptoms depend on the region deprived of flow
- CVA or Stroke: It rapidly developing clinical symptoms and signs of focal and at times global loss of cerebral function, with symptoms lasting more than 24 hours with no apparent cause other than that of vascular origin (Hatano 1976).

## RISK FACTORS

- Hypertension
- Cardiac disease
- Age
- Gender (Male/Female)
- Diabetes Mellitus
- Family History
- Smoking
- Alcohol
- Increased hematocrit
- TIA
- Elevated fibrinogen level
- Hemoglobinopathy.

## PATHOPHYSIOLOGY

- Cerebral Ischemia defined as the degree and duration of blood flow loss, largely determines whether the brain suffers only temporary dysfunction, irreversible injury to a few highly neurons (Ischemic necrosis) or damage to extensive areas involving all cell types (cerebral infarction)
- A failed delivery of oxygen and glucose to the brain
- Cerebral Infarction: irreversible cellular damage
- Cerebral Edema: Increases in the water content of the brain (edema) accompany all types of ischemic and hemorrhagic strokes
- Brain swelling and raised intracranial pressure.

## CLINICAL NEUROVASCULAR SYMPTOMS

| Table: 4.1: Features of the Stroke | |
|---|---|
| *Ischemic Stroke* | *Symptoms* |
| Internal Cartoid artery | Ipsilateral Blindness<br>MCA Syndrome |
| Middle Cerbral artery (MCA) | Contralateral Hemiparesis<br>Sensory loss (arm, face, worst)<br>Expressive aphasia (Dominant)<br>Anosognosia and spatial disorientation (nondominant) |
| Anterior cerebral artery | Contralateral hemiparesis<br>Sensory loss (worst in leg) |
| Posterior cerebral artery | Contralateral homonymous hemianopsia or<br>Superior quadrantanopsia<br>· Memory impairment |
| Basilar Apex | Bilateral blindness, Amnesia |
| Basilar artery | Contralateral hemiparesis,<br>Sensory loss<br>Ipsilateral bulbar or cerebellar signs |
| Vertebral artery of Posterior Inferior cerebellar artery | Ipsilateral loss of facial sensation<br>Ataxia<br>Contralateral hemiparesis<br>Sensory loss |
| Superior cerebellar artery | Gait ataxia |
| | Nausea<br>Dizziness<br>Headach<br>Progressing to ipsilateral hemiataxia<br>Dysarthria<br>Gaze paresis, Contralateral hemiparesis. |

### Laboratory Investigations

*Hematology*

- Complete blood count, glucose, prothrombin times, partial thromboplastin time, lipid profile, electrolytes, creatinine, blood

urea nitrogen, protein, and erythrocyte sedimentation rate should be performed
- Tests of renal function and serum electrolyte measurements.

## Cardiovascular Tests

- 12 Lead (ECG) Electrocardiogram—to evaluate acute myocardial ischemia and arrhythmias.
- Echocardiography—for cardiogenic source of emboli in acute stroke.
- Stress Testing—to evaluate possible ischemic cardiovascular disease.

## Radiodiagnostic Imaging

### CT Scan Imaging

- To identify other causes of focal neurologic dysfunction such as neoplasms or subdural hematomas and to distinguish ischemic from hemorrhagic stroke
- Can be used to evaluate CSF space, brain tissue perfusion.

### MRI Scan Imaging

- Imaging for blood vessels, blood flow and smaller lesion (Lacunar strokes, cerebral infarction)
- Acute infarctions (with in first 24 hours).

### Lumbar Puncture

- Diagnosing neurosyphils or meningitis.

### Cerebral Angiography

- Intracranial and extracranial cerebral angiography of elderly patients to ischemic stroke
- Cerebral angiography should be reserved for specific indications (e.g. for fibromuscular dysplasia, arterial dissection, and cranial arteritis).

## Other Techniques

### Positron Emission Tomography (PET)

- Using radiolabeled water or carbon dioxide
- For imaging cerebral blood flow, brain metabolism.

### Single Photon Emission computed Tomography (SPECT)

*Doppler sonography and Quantitative Ocular pneumoplethysmography:*
- Help to evaluate the cerbrovascular supply
- Direct examination of the common internal and external carotid arteries is best achieved by Doppler sonography
- To measure the frequency shift associated with increased blood velocity through a stenotic lumen.

## STROKE ASSESSMENT

- Observe for signs of increased intracranial pressure
- Assess level of consciousness and cognitive function
- Assess speech and communication
  - Aphasia
  - Perceptual deficits.

## Assess Changes in Behavior

### Assess sensory deficits

- Superficial, Proprioceptive and combined sensations of contra lateral extremities and trunk, face.

### Assess Hearing

- Vision, check for homonymous hemianopsia.

### Assess Cranial Nerves

- Seventh cranial nerve involvement
- Vertebro basilar stroke (Pseudobulbar palsy).

## Assess Motor System

- Presence of abnormal muscle tone
- Primitive reflexes
- Loss of selective movements
- Presences of basic limb synergies
- Upper limb flexion synergy: Scapula retraction/elevation, shoulder abduction, external rotation, elbow flexion, forearm supination, wrist and flexion
- Upper limb extension synergy: scapular protraction, shoulder abduction, internal rotation, elbow extension, forearm pronation, wrist and finger flexion
- Lower extremity flexion synergy: Hip flexion, abduction, external rotation, knee flexion, ankle doriflexion and inversion
- Lower extremity extension synergy: Hip extension, abduction, internal rotation, knee extension, ankle plantar flexion and inversion
- Presence of paresis of muscles.

## Assess Coordination

- Finger to finger, heel to shin, supination, pronation test, finger to nose, Romberg's sign.

## Postural Control and Balance

- Using Posturography, Berg Balance scale (0 -4).

## Gait

- Circumduction gait or Hemiplegic gait,
- Equines gait,
- Unstable step lengths,
- Cadence,
- Insufficent pelvic rotation during swing,
- Weak hip flexors (external rotation with adduction, backward leaning of trunk).

## Assess ADLs

- Barthel Index, Functional mobility skills (FMS).

## Stroke Assessment Tools/ Scales

*Motor Assessment scales (MAS) (Carr. et al. 1979)*

- Measures functional capabilities, using 8 categories of movements.

*Bobath*

- Evaluation of motor patterns, qualitive assessment of movement and postural patterns
- Based on three main recovery stage:
  - Flaccidity stage
  - Spasticity stage
  - Stage of relative recovery.

## OTHER IMPAIRMENT OF STROKE SCALES

- Brunstrom - Fugl meyer Assessement
- Chedoke Mcmaster stroke
- Storke assessement sot
- Toronto stroke scale
- Mathew stroke scale
- National Institute of Health stroke scale
- Canadian neurological scale, and
- Orgogozo score and Hemispheric stroke scale.

## PHYSICAL THERAPY INTERVENTION

### Acute Stroke

- About 10-15% of patients with stroke die, because of brain swelling or neurologic dysfunction (impaired respiration with medullary infarctions, myocardial infarction, pulmonary embolus and pneumonia).

### Aims

*Improve / Maintain Normal Oxygen and Ventilation*

- Clearance of airways
- Improve chest expansion

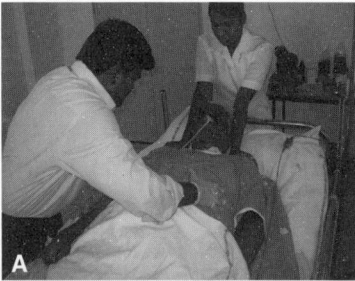

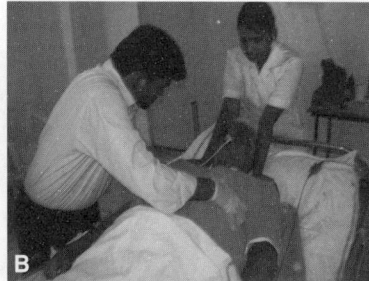

**Figs 4.1A and B:** Assisted Coughing

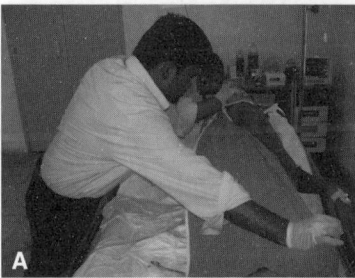

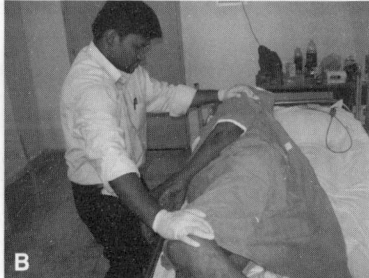

**Figs 4.2A and B:** Rolling in bed to sound side

- Removal of secretions
- Improve cough effectiveness (Fig. 4.1)
- Improve breathing pattern/breathing sounds
- Prevent bed sores (Fig. 4.2).

*Improve/ Maintain Musculoskeletal System within Functional Limit*

- Improve range of motion (ROM) (Fig. 4.3)
- Improve muscle strength and Endurance
- Prevent joint deformities and contractures (Fig. 4.4A and B).

*Improve Circulatory System Function*

- Prevent Deep Vein Thrombosis (DVT)
- Prevent swelling.

Stroke Physical Therapy

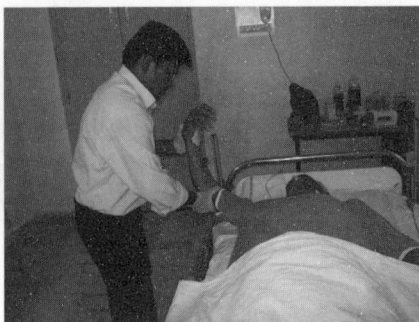

**Fig.: 4.3** Passive ROM exercise to right shoulder joint

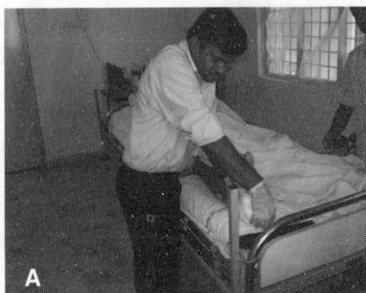

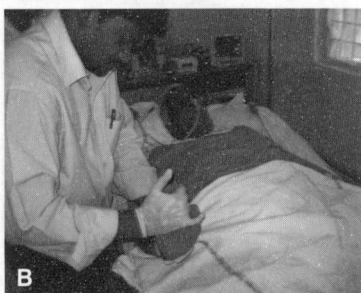

**Figs 4.4 A and B:** Stretching: (A) To right dorsiflexors of the ankle.
(B) Stretching right wrist flexors

## Pulmonary Dysfunction/Care

- Regular and Frequent turning
- Chest physical therapy techniques of Percussion, Vibration, shaking and rib springing to the chest
- Postural drainage
- Mechanical suction
- Positioning.

## Musculoskeletal Problems

- Passive ROM exercise should be started at the early stage of stroke
- Use to prevent contractures, improving circulation and preventing stiffness
- Avoid overstretching of soft tissue musculature and impingement at glenohumeral joint, particularly in acute stage of stroke.

Stroke Physical Therapy

## Positioning (Figs 4.5A and B)

- Positioning refers to the application of body positioning to optimize oxygen transport, primarily by manipulating the effect of gravity on cardiopulmonary and cardiovascular disease (Elizabeth D, 2005)
- The aim of routine positioning is primarily to reduce the adverse effects of restricted mobility including pulmonary complications (e.g. Pneumonia), bed sores and contractures
- To prevent development of abnormal posture, spasticity and contractures (head, trunk and limbs should be maintained (Nair, KPS, 2002)
- The frequent turning of a patient will not only benefit the musculoskeletal system and aid pressure relief, but will also enhance the respiratory system.

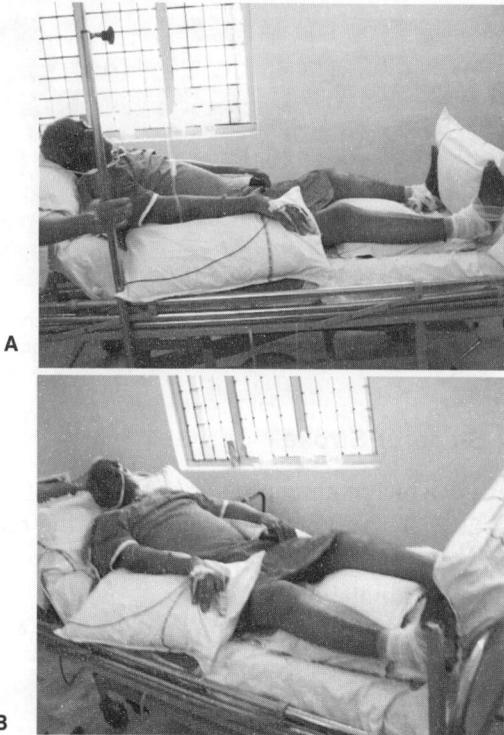

A

B

**Figs 4.5 A and B:** Positioning a critically ill patient may require several people and continual monitoring of the patient's response

Stroke Physical Therapy

## Active Exercises

- Should be instituted as soon as the person is conscious (Carr.J, 2004)
- Active Assisted Arm exercise: Increase muscle tone and range of motion (Figs 4.6 A to D).

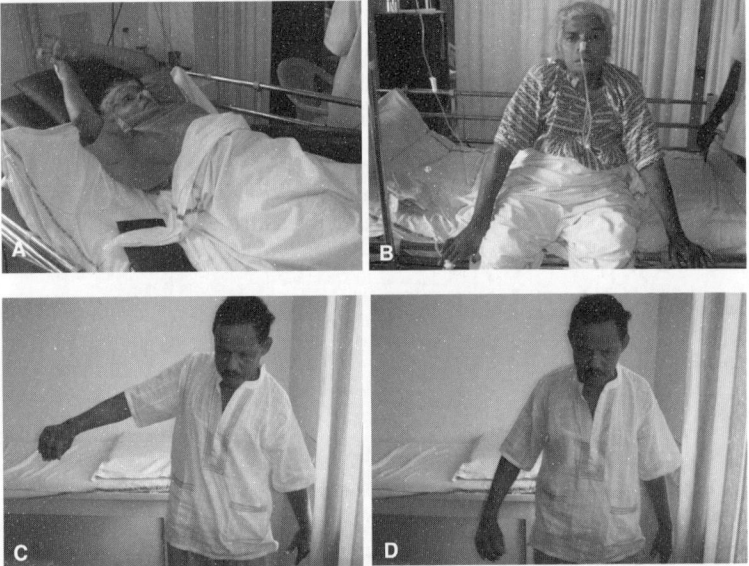

**Figs 4.6 A to D:** (A) Active Assisted Arm Exercise (B) Patient is able to sit independently   (C) and (D) Active ROM exercise (Abduction)

## Recovery Stage of Stroke

- The Period which commences once the patient is medically stable, conscious and actively engaged in the rehabilitation process
- The aim of Rehabilitation is:
  - Prevent secondary emotional, intellectual and physical deterioration
  - Prevent complications of immobilization
  - Improve ADLs, skills.

## Task Related Training

- The patient can practice independently, should be identified to involve the patient as an active participant in his /her own rehabilitation (Ada and Canning, 1990).

## Motor Learning Techniques (MLT)

- Motor learning techniques (MLT)–is to used for encouraging learning, include goal identification, instruction, auditory and visual feedback, manual guidance and practice.

## Bobath/NDT Techniques

*Brunnstrom Method*

Weight bearing exercise– to strengthen lower limb extensors.
Steeping exercise– to improve walking.

## Functional Mobility Training (Figs 4.7A to F)

- Rolling, supine to sit, sitting (Fig. 4.8), sit to stand, transfers (Fig. 4.8), wheelchair mobility and ambulation (O' Sullivan. S, 2005).

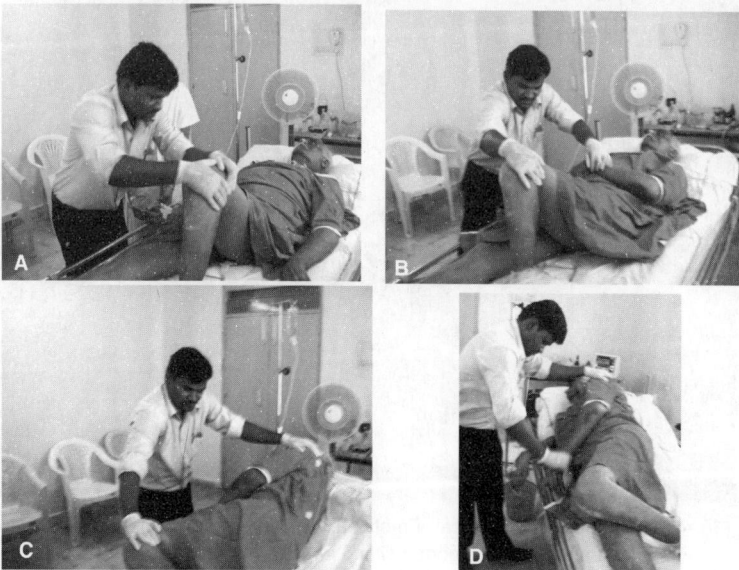

Figs 4.7 A to D:

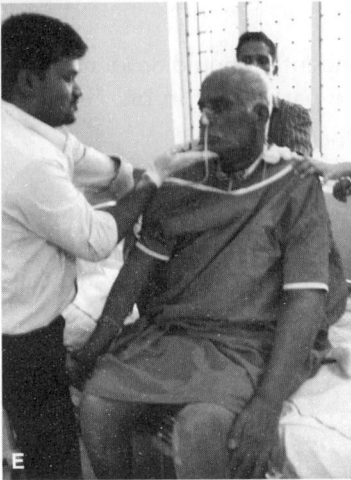

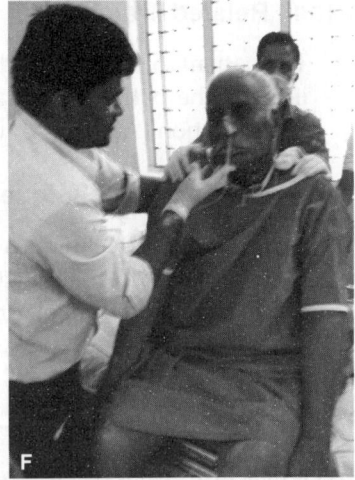

**Figs 4.7 E to F:** Progressive transfer supine from supine lying to sitting on the edge of bed

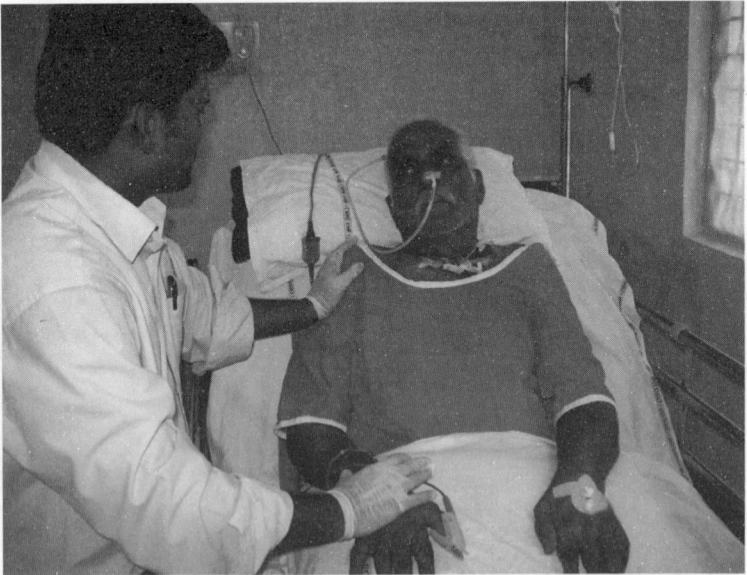

**Fig. 4.8:** Patients Psychological, Emotional support and motivation by physical therapist, and supported sitting in bed placed on a pillow

## ACTIVITIES OF DAILY LIVING (ADLS) SKILLS

- To regain functional independence of activities of daily living (Figs 4.9A to D)
- Use of arm and hand in simple tasks such as dressing is the best way to facilitate motor recovery
- Patient can be taught hemiparetic dressing technique, which begins on hemiplegic side first
- Self feeding can be helped with the use of friction plates, rocker knives and other modified utensils.

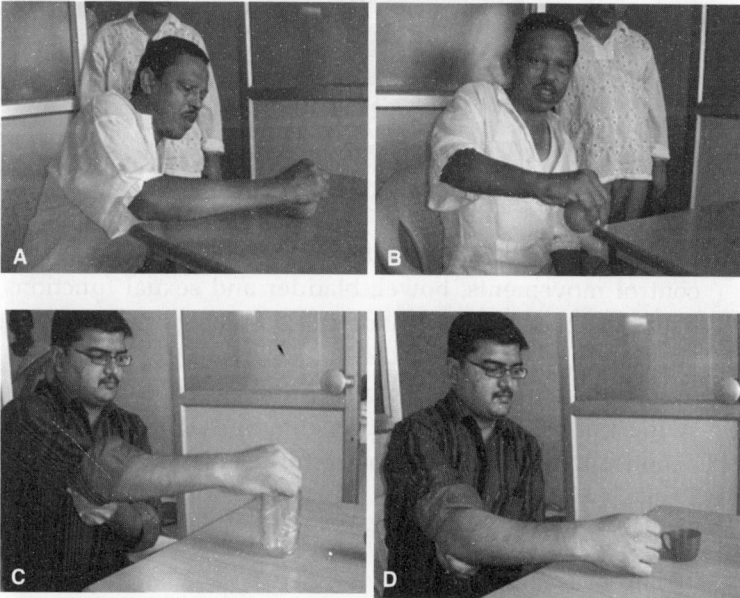

**Figs 4.9 A to D:** Post Stroke: Weakness of Hand muscles (A) and (B). He is Difficult to hold and manipulate objects, i. e, wrist extension and forearm Supination are absent. (C) and (D) Reaching is attempted. He attempts to reach the object in paralysed or weak hand muscles

### Exercise Conditioning

- Cycle Ergometry (Fig. 4.10)
- Walking

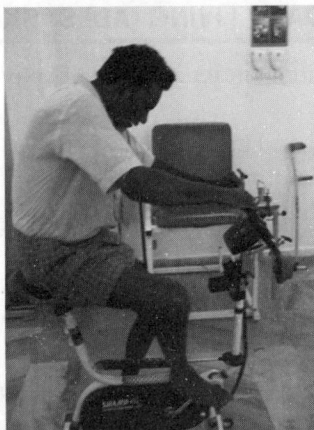

**Fig. 4.10:** Bicycle ergometer training

## Recent Physical Therapy Training Modes

### Functional Electrical Stimulation

- These techniques can be used to improve the muscle strength, control movements, bowel, bladder and sexual functions, maintenance of posture, standing and walking (Maxwell OJ, et al 1995)
- Indication: Peroneal nerve stimulation to correct foot drop during swing phase of gait. This prevents muscle atrophy, bone demineralization and joint contractures.

### EMG Biofeedback

- To improve motor functions
- Useful to strengthening Tibialis anterior, Quadriceps, Hamstrings and upper extremity muscles
- EMG initiated electrical stimulation to improve arm and hand functions in chronic hemiplegia (Kraft GH, et al 1992).

### Body weight–Supported Treadmill Training (BWSTT)

- Hesse and colleagues (1994) examined the effects of treadmill walking on nine patients who could not at all or required the assistance of minutes per session and within 5 days they had increased this time to 30 minutes

Stroke Physical Therapy

- Slow treadmill speeds (typically 0.01 -2.25 m/s) and light support using an over head harness (typically 30% of body weight to start) are used
- One or two Physical therapists provide manual assistance in stabilization of trunk/pelvis and in movement of the paretic limb.

*Kinetron for Reciprocal Stepping motions – to improve the gait*

*Isokinetic Training*

- Use to increase strength and velocity control of movement.

*Constraint – Induced Therapy (CIT)*

*Robot – Assisted Movement Therapy (RAMT)*

## Orthotics Devices

- The use of orthoses following stroke is to lengthen shortened soft tissue
- Serial Casting: To improve functional performance and lengthen soft tissues
- Ankle foot orthoses (AFO) (Fig. 4.11):
  - Rigid and Hinged type of orthosis
  - To stabilize an ankle by preventing excessive inversion of the foot

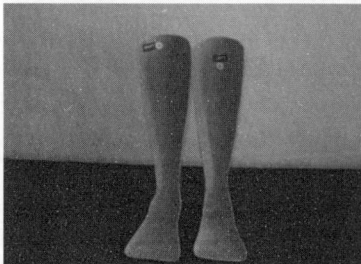

**Fig. 4.11:** Ankle -Foot- Orthosis (AFO)     **Fig. 4.12:** Wrist Cock up Splint

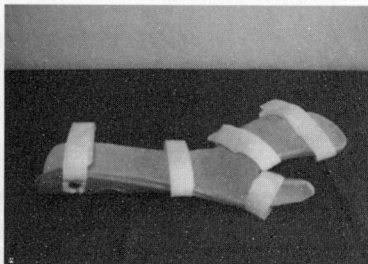

- Upper extremity resting hand splints are used to prevent deformity and to maintain the hemiplegic wrist in a functional, slightly extended position (Delisa JA, 2005) (Fig. 4.12)
- Strapping or Splint: It can be used to alter the direction of the movements of the muscles pull or prevent adaptive movements at the glenohumeral joint.

## Mobility Aids

- Wheel Chair: It is to promote early independence
- Walking aids: Quadripod cane, walker, Parallel bars, Cane or stick (Fig. 4.13A and B) are frequently used for individuals with poor balance and additional support through the lower limbs during standing and walking.

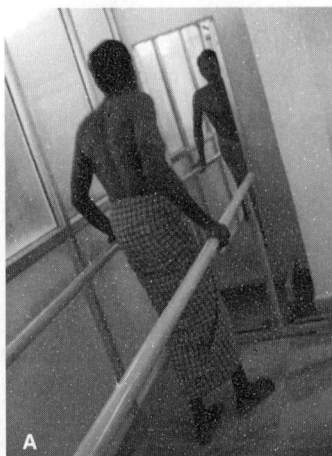

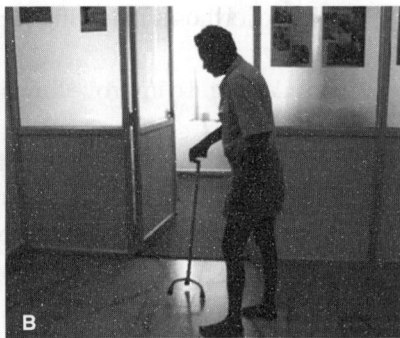

**Figs 4.13A and B:** Parallel bar training; He is able to walk with cane support

## Complications of Stroke

- Immobility related complications are very common in the first year in a severely disabling stroke. Patients who are more frequently dependent at 3 months post stroke are likely to experience a greater number of complications than those are less dependent (sackley C, et al. 2008). These complications include; shoulder pain, shoulder hand syndrome, pressure sores, contracture, deep vein thrombosis, shoulder pain

- If patient localized discomfort to any aspect of the affected shoulder when assessed by the Physiotherapist
- Shoulder pain and stiffness impede the rehabilitation of patients with hemiplegia
- The cause of this complication is unknown, but it may be related to the severity of neurologic deficits, preexisting or post hemiplegic soft tissue injury, subluxation, brachial plexus injury or shoulder hand syndrome. Shoulder pain may be preventable if risk factors identified and appropriate prophylaxis applied (Judy WG, 1986).

## Shoulder Hand Syndrome (SHS)

- Shoulder hand syndrome were originally described by "Stein brocker"
- Pain in the hemiplegic arm may in some cases be constellation of symptoms, often referred to as the shoulder hand syndrome or Reflex sympathetic dystrophy
- The incidence 12.5% of the undiagnosed condition may be much larger
- The syndrome can occur in patients whose upper limbs are flaccid and without contractures
- Symptoms: Edema of wrist, MCP, and PIP. Hot, dry and red or blotchy skin, Severe pain in the hand or shoulder or both and protectively restricts any movement or sensory input to the limb
- Gradually, muscle atrophy and trophic changes in skin, connective tissue and joints
- A typical deformity of hand is metacarpal joint extension and IP joints flexion, resembling the "Intrinsic Minus Hand".

## Investigations

- X-rays, MRI and Bone scan.

## Physical Therapy Treatment

- Vigorous painful stretching of the affected shoulder should be avoided

- Proper handling techniques
- Passive or assistive elevation is used to reduce spasticity
- Scapular mobilization and Humeral external rotation
- Bobath, Johnstone and Brunnstrom approaches
- Avoid shoulder pulleys and Pasive elevation of the affected arm.

## Shoulder Glenuohumeral Joint (GHJ) Subluxation

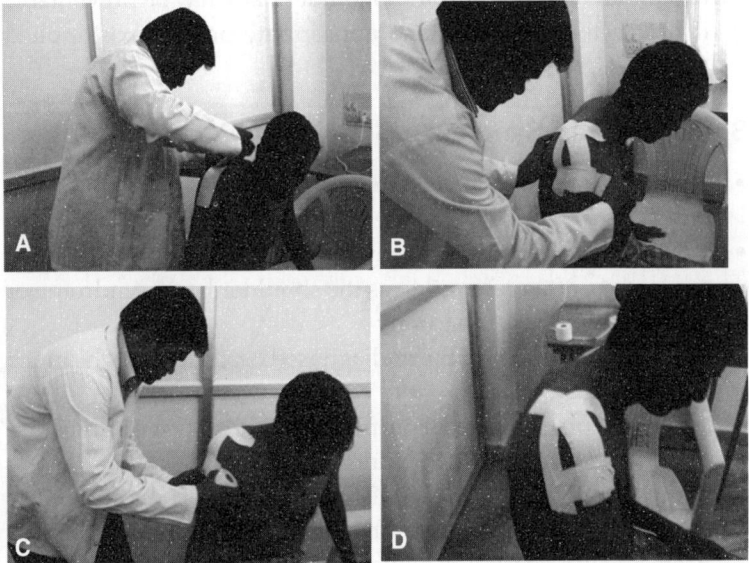

**Figs 4.14A to D:** Shoulder strapping

## Treatment

- To prevent GHJ subluxation in the first few weeks after onset of hemiplegia
- Shoulder slings is use to prevent shoulder subluxation
- Immobilization of arms
- Positioning
- Strapping (Figs 4.14A to D)
- EMG Biofeedback
- Active range of motion exercise(AROM)
- Cryotherapy
- Functional Electrical stimulation (FES)
- Postural support

## Pressure Sores (Figs 4.15A to C)

- Areas of localized damage to the skin and underlying tissue caused by pressure, shear or friction were considered pressure sores. Identification was based on physical examination
- Pressure sores are common in elderly, undernourished and immobile stroke patient.

### Incidence

7.7 % of hospitalized patients develops pressure ulcers within 21 days of admission.

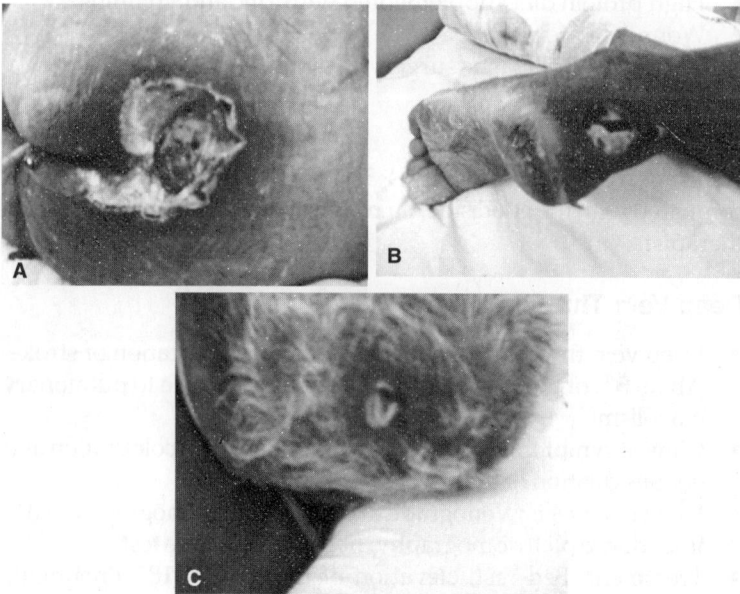

**Figs 4.15A to C:** Pressure sores: (A) Sacrum (B) Calcaneum (C) Occipital

### Various stages

- Stage I – Non blanchable erthema of intact skin.
- Stage II – Partial Thickness skin loss.
- Stage III – Full thickness skin loss.
- Stage IV – Extension into muscles and bones.

### Common Pressure Points

Lateral malleolus, Sacrum, Coccyx, Greater trochanter, calcaneum. Occipital region.

*Prevention*

- Avoid continuous pressure over bony prominences
- Changing the position once every two hours
- Avoiding friction and moisture over the skin
- Proper positioning of the limbs using sand bags.

*Treatment*

- Pressure relieving surfaces like water bed or alternating pressure mattress
- Anterior, lateral, and press- up weight shifting techniques
- High protein diet supplemented with zinc and vitamins
- Wound débridement
- Antibotics and Plastic surgery.

## Contracture

Contracture was estimated as 30% or higher restriction when compared with the good side, on physical examination by a Physical therapist.

## Deep Vein Thrombosis (DVT)

- Deep vein thrombosis is major medical complication of stroke. About 5% of the deaths in stroke patients are due to pulmonary embolism
- Clinical symptoms: Pain, tenderness, edema, discolouration and venous dilation of the affected extremity
- Diagnostic tests: Venography, doppler ultrasonography, MRI, impedance plethsomography, fibrinogen uptake test
- Treatment: Bed rest, elevation of the foot by 18", Pneumatic Intermittent compression of calf muscles of the paretic leg, free toe movements, compression stockings.

## Effects of Stroke on Family

- Survivors from stroke depend on their family members for emotional and physical support. About 34-52 % of care givers of patients with stroke suffer from depression. Psychosocial therapy should be started with family members at the time of the patient's hospitalization and begin with patient as soon as possible.

Stroke Physical Therapy

- The family member who is closest to the patient and practice under supervision of a Physical therapist. Family members should provide encouragement, show confidence in improvement and permit the recovering person to do as much he or she can and to be as independent and vigorous as possible.

## BIBLIOGRAPHY

- Anchlifee J. Strapping the shoulder in patients following a Cerebrovascular Accident: A pilot study. Australian J Physiotherapy, 38(1), 37- 491.
- Anthony J, Zollo JR. Medical Secrets, Elsevier sciences, Philadelphia, 2006;475-98.
- Carr j, Shwpard R. Neuro Rehabilitation. 2nd ed Woburn MA, Butterworth- Heineman 1998.
- Caillet R. The shoulder in Hemiplegia. FA Davis; Philladelphia, 1980.
- Chaudhuri JR, Taly TB. Neuro Rehabilitation: Concepts and Dynamics in Neuro Rehabilitation; Prinicples and practice. Ahuja Book Company, Bangalore, 2001; p. 38-48.
- Christopher MB, Catherine SM. Manual of Physical medicine and Rehabilitation, Elsevier, Hanley and Belfus, Inc, 2002; 281-96.
- Dobkin BH. Stroke Rehabilitation, FA Davis, Philadelphia, 1996;157-217.
- Dromerick A, Reding M. Medical and Neurological Complications during inpatient Stroke Rehabilitation. Stroke, 1994;25: 358-61.
- Diane UJ, et al. Physical therapy interventions for patients with stroke inpatient Rehabilitation facilities. APTA J; Jan 2005; 157-217.
- Dickstein R, Hocherman S, Pillar T, et al. Stroke Rehabilitation three Exercise therapy Approaches, Phys Ther 1986;66:1233-38.
- David OW,Valery LF, Robert DB. Hand Book of Stroke, 2nd ed, Lippincott wiliams and wilkins 2006.
- Ernst E. A Review of Stroke Rehabilitation and Physiotherapy Stroke, 1990;21:1081-85.
- Evens RL, Hendricks Rd, Haselkorn JK, et al. The Family role in Stroke Rehabilitation; A Review of the literature. Am J. Phys Med Rehabilitation, 1992; 71:135-9.
- Edwards S. Neurological Physical therapy; A problem solving Approach, London, Churchill Livingstone, 1996.
- Franceschini M, Carda S, Agosti M, et al. Walking after Stroke: What does Treadmill Training with Body Weight Support Add to Overground Gait Training in patients Early After Stroke? A Single Blind, randomized, controlled trial, Stroke, 2009;40: 3079-85.
- Gibbons B. Stroke Rehabilitation, Nurs. Stand, 1994;8:49-54.
- Hesse S, Bertelt C, Jahnke MT, et al. Treadmill training with partial weight support compared with Physiotherapy in nonambulatory Hemiparetic patients stroke, 1995;26:976-81.

- Hidler H, Nicholes D, Pelliccio M, Brady K, Campbell DD, et al. Multicenter randomized clinical trial evaluating the effectiveness of the Lokmat in subacute stroke. Neurorehabilitation neural repair, 2009;23: 5-13.
- Harrison MA. Physical therapy in Stroke Rehabilitation, Churchill Livingstone, Newyork, 1995; 57-62.
- Intiso D, Santilli V, Grasso MG, et al. Rehabilitation of Walking with Electromyographic Biofeedback in foot drop after stroke. Stroke, 1994; 25:1189-92.
- Jette DU, Brown R, Collette N, et al. Physical therapists management of Patients in the Acute care setting: An observational study. Phys Ther 2009; 89(11):1158-81.
- Judy WG. Hemiplegic Shoulder Pain, Phys Ther 1986, Vol: 66; NO:12; PP: 1884-93.
- Jette DU, Latham NK, Smout RJ, Gassaway J, Slavin MD, Hom SD. Physical therapy interventions for patients with stroke inpatient rehabilitation facilities. Phys Ther, 2005; 85(3): 238-48.
- Judy G, Gay R. Shoulder Pain in Patients with Hemiplegia. A Literature Review. Phys Ther 1981; vol 61 (no): 7, July.
- Klotz T, Borges HC, Montero VC, Chamlian TR, Masiero P. Physiotherapy Treatment in Hemiplegic Shoulder Pain in Stroke Patients - Literature Review, ACTA FISIATR, 2006;13(11):12-6.
- Lyden PP, Hantson L. Assessment Scales for the evaluation of stroke patients. J. Stroke Cerebrovascular Accident Diseases, 1998;7: 113-27.
- Langton Hewer R. Rehabilitation after Stroke, QJM, 1990; 76:659-74.
- Maxwell DJ, ferguson ACB, Granat MH, et al. Functional electrical stimulation in stroke rehabilitation. In Physiotherapy in stroke Management, Harrison MA (Ed), Churchill Livingstone, New York, 1995; 57-62.
- Maklebust J, Sieggreen M. Pressure Ulcers: Guidelines for prevention and management, 3rd springhouse, PA, Springhouse corp, 2001.
- Michael D. Brain's Disease of the nervous system. Stroke , p. 775-896.
- Mant J, Carter J, Wade DT, et al. Family support for stroke; A randomized controlled trial, Lancet, 2000; 356; 808-13.
- Nawoczenski D, Epler M. Orthosis in functional rehabilitation of the lower limb. Philadelphia, WB Saunders Co.
- Nair, KPS, Taly AB. Stroke Rehabilitation; Traditional and Modern Approaches. NeuroIndia, vol. 50, Dec 2002; PP; S85-S93.
- Stephen JM, Papadakis MA. Large current medical diagnosis and treatment, 4th ed, Mc-Graw Hill, 2009.
- The Cochrane Database of syst. Review. Overground Physical therapy Gait training for people with Chronic Stroke with mobility deficits. Art, No: CD oo6075, 2009.
- Umphered D (ed) - Neurological Rehabilitation. 4th ed, St.Louis, CV Mosby, 2004.
- Wild D. Stroke Focus, Stroke: A Nursing Rehabilitation role. Nurs. Stand, 1994;8:36-9.
- Wade DT, et al. Physiotherapy intervention late after Stroke and mobility, BMJ, 2009;13: 304-609.

# Chapter

## 5

# Physical Therapy in Muscular Dystrophy

## MUSCULAR DYSTROPHY

- Muscular Dystrophy is a group of genetic diseases marked by progressive muscle weakness and degeneration of the skeletal or voluntary muscles, which control movement. Age at onset and inheritance pattern depend on the specific dystrophy.

## CLASSIFICATION

- Duchenne type
- Becker
- Limb girdle (Erb)
- Facioscapulohumeral
- Emery-Dreifus
- Distal
- Ocular
- Oculopharyngeal
- Myotonic dystrophy.

### Duchenne Muscular Dystrophy (DMD)

- Duchenne muscular dystrophy is a X-linked recessive, genetic, neuro muscular disease. It is caused by a problem with gene that makes a protein called dystrophin. The affected gene codes for the protein dystrophin, which is markedly reduced or absent from the muscles of patients with the disease.

### Incidence

- The disease is inherited; males are likely to develop symptoms than are women. Approximately one out of every 3,600 male infants.
- Age at onset 1 to 5 years.

### Pathology

- An absence of defect in the protein dystrophin (Xp21-2) which results in progressive muscle degeneration leading to loss of independent ambulation by the age of 13 years

- Collagen, adipose laid down in muscle leading to pseudo hypertrophic calf muscles.

## Clinical Manifestations

- Motor milestones delay
- Delayed walking
- Hypotonia
- Climbing stairs, rising from the ground after falling
- Positive Gower's sign – is always present, with boys needing to turn on to their front and rise to standing from the floor using a broad based stance, usually with the support of their hands on their thighs (Figs 5.1A to F)
- Pelvic girdle muscle weakness
- Lordotic posture
- Trendlenburg gait or Waddling gait
- Weakness of musculature of the calf, Gluetal vastus lateralis, Deltoid and Infraspinatus groups
- Tendon reflexes are diminshed at the knees, biceps and triceps
- Contractures: Tendo-Achilles, Hamstrings, iliotibial band, Hip flexors, Elbow flexors, Forearm pronators, Long finger flexors
- Thoracic deformity: Scoliosis
- Enlargement of calves (Pseudohypertrophy and wasting of thigh muscles). The enlargement is caused by hypertrophy of some muscle fibers, infiltration of muscle by fat and proliferation of collagen
- Muscular hypertrophy of the tongue
- Pharyngeal weakness
- Cardiomyopathy
- Intellectual impairment
- Myalgia and muscle spasm do not occur
- Dealth, usually at about 18 years of age. The cause of death are respiratory failure in sleep, intractable heart failure, pneumonia or aspiration and airway obstruction.

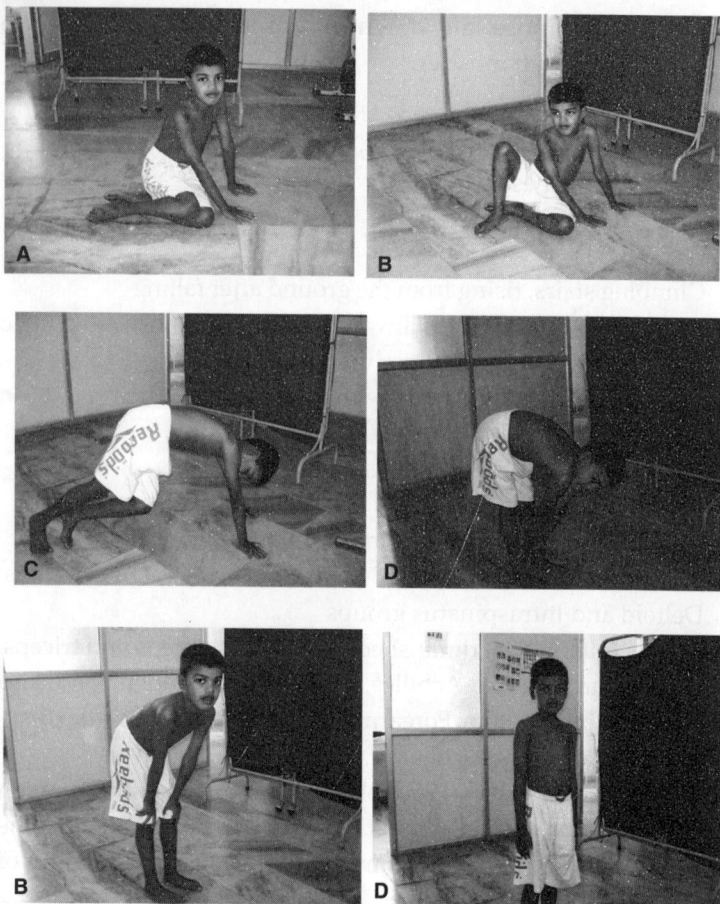

Figs 5.1A to F: Gower's maneuver

## Diagnosis

### Laboratory Findings

- **Serum Creatine kinase Level** is elevated in Duchenne muscular dystrophy. The usual serum concentration is 15,000 - 35,000 IU/L (Normal < 160 IU/L)
- **Electrocardiography (ECG),** Echocardiography and Chest roentenogram - for assessment of heart

- **Electromyography (EMG):** Shows distinctively myopathic, with decreases seen in the amplitude and duration of the compound action potential and enrichment of the interference pattern
- **Sensory and Motor Nerve Conduction Velocity:** Help to determine if the disorder lies in the anterior horn cell, the peripheral or the muscle
- **Muscle Biopsy** is usually required to confirm the diagnosis (Bertorini et al. 2002). The muscle histology demonstrates dystrophic features which include an increased varation of fiber size, evidence of necrosis with phagocytosis, an increase in central nuclei, hypercontracted eosinophillic hyaline fibers and an increase in fat and connective tissue (Thompson N and Quinlivan 2004). The most common muscles sampled are the vastus lateralis (Quadriceps femoris) and the gastrocnemius
- **Deoxyribonucleic acid (DNA) Testing:** Findings of a DNA deletion, duplication or point mutation allows carrier detection and prenatal diagnosis in the affected boy's mother and female relatives. In some cases DNA analysis is the only test required to conform the diagnosis of DMD.

## Assessment

- Regular assessment of child with DMD is most essential because they change rapidly. The Clinical evaluation and measurement of muscle strength, range of motion, posture, functional performance, alignment, gait and lung function.

## Measurement of Muscle Strength

- Medical research Council (MRC) Scale: Grading of 0-5.
- Other methods: Dynamometry (Hyde, et al. 1983), myometry (Bohannon 1986).

## Joint Range of Motion (ROM)

- Active joint movements can be measured using goniometry (Pandya et al. 1985).

## Measurement of Functional Performance

- Measures of functional performance range from simple tests, such as the ability to rise from the floor (Rideau, 1984)
- Hammersmith score of motor ability (Score 2, 1 or 0)
- Vignos Scale was assessment of functional ability in progressive neuromuscular conditions.

## Timed Tests

- Timed performance tests was used to measures of physical performance (progressive weakness in children with DMD)
- Measure to walking speed , distance and to get up from the floor.

## Lung function tests: Spirometry

## PHYSICAL THERAPY INTERVENTION

## Aims

- To maintain physical function for as long as possible
- Prevent disabling consequences of secondary problems
- Physical therapists provide guidance support
- Education about condition
- Advocacy–insurers, schools and providers of recreation.

Physical Therapy input is essential for the maintance of muscle function in Duchenne muscular dystrophy. Initially the priority is the maintenance of symmetry as development of asymmetric contractures at the achilles tendon and hip's can predispose to pelvic obliquity and subsequent scoliosis.

## Passive Stretching

- Tendo-achilles, Hamstrings, Iliotibial band, Iliopsoas, Later shoulders, elbow, wrist muscles will need to stretched (Figs 5.2 and 5.3) and prevented for development of contractures.

Physical Therapy in Muscular Dystrophy

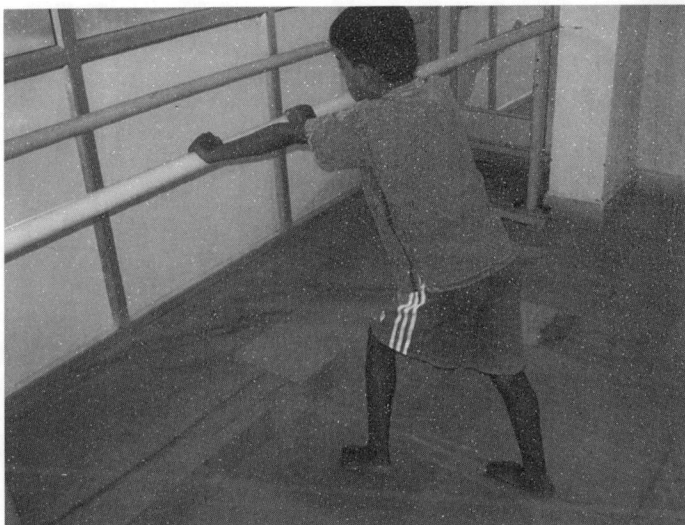

**Fig. 5.2:** Active stretching exercise (Calf Muscles)

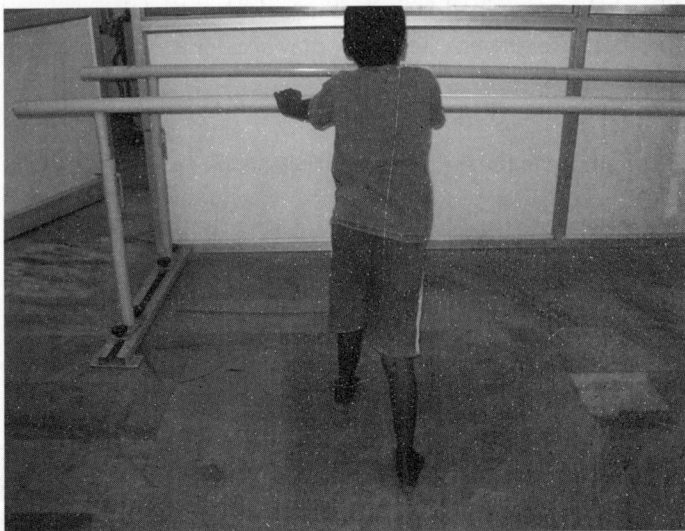

**Fig. 5.3:** Right side calf muscle stretching

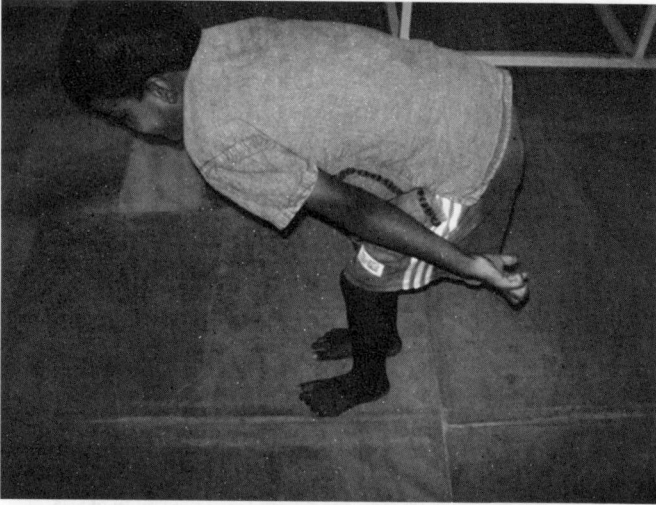

**Fig. 5.4:** Active trunk flexion/extension exercise

### Resisted Exercise

• Should be prescribed as there is no evidence that they are useful but there are concerns that they may accelerate muscle damage.

### Active Exercise (Fig. 5.4)

• Particularly in the hydrotherapy pool is recommend

### Motor Skills Training

• Such as riding a bike and this encourages independent play and interaction with peers.

### Ankle Foot Orthoses (AFOs)

• At night these are the mainstay of treatment ambulant stage to delay development of contractures, together with encouragement to be active and take part in sports other activities as hydro therapy and appropriate physical educational school.

**Physical Therapy in Muscular Dystrophy**

## Knee Ankle Foot Orthoses (KAFOs)

- Also known as long leg calipers
- May be considered to prolong the ability to walk and stand around the time ambulation is lost. The use of long leg calipers rarely allows the achievement of independent ambulation.

## Special Seating and Head Support

- Should be introduced early before there are detrimental postural adaptations.

## WHEELCHAIR OR NONAMBULANT CHILDREN

## Management

- Sitting AFOs are essential as painful contractures will develop, that also impact negatively on posture
- Passive or active assisted exercise should be continued for comfort, aesthetics and contracture prevention
- Pressure sores from sever contractures should be avoided
- Surgery: Triple arthrodesis may required in children who develop severe deformity of the ankle
- Wheelchairs: It should be supplied to improve mobility and independence
- Tilt-in-Space electric wheelchairs with supporting seating should be supplied early to avoid postural contractures and poor sitting posture.

## PREVENTION AND MANAGEMENT OF SPINAL DEFORMITY

## Aim

- Preventing further deformity
- Promoting better seating posture and comfort
- 90% of boys with Duchenne muscular dystrophy are likely to develop a clinically significant scoliosis

- Provision of proper seating to prevent pelvic asymmetry and provide postural support
- Spinal Bracing: Provides comfort and postural security in children who are unable to have spinal surgery
- A Light weight polypropylene Thoraco - Lumbar-Sacral Orthosis (TLSO)– to prevent lumber lordosis and scoliosis.

## RESPIRATORY MANAGEMENT IN DMD

### Problems

- Loss of respiratory muscle strength
- Ineffective cough and decreased ventilation
- Pneumonia
- Atelectasis and respiratory insufficiency.

## AIM: TO PREVENT RESPIRATORY COMPLICATIONS AND CHEST INFECTION

### Treatment

- Chest physical therapy
- Breathing exercise
- Percussion of the chest
- Postural drainage
- Assisted coughing techniques
- Use of glossopharyngeal breathing (In essence forcing air into the lungs using one's mouth)
- Spirometry
- Air stacking
- Mechanical assisted ventilation or mechanical assisted airway clearance therapy.

### Associated Problems

*Bone Health*

- Low bone mineral density even before loss of independent

ambulation. This may relate to their relative immobility even at early stages of the disease
- Long bone fractures are common
- Aim: Reduces bone mineral density further
- Treatment: Calicum and vitamin D intake through diet and sunshine with supplementation (Quinlivan R 2005).

## BIBLIOGRAPHY

- Bakker JDJ, Groot I, Beckerman, Dejong, Lankhorst GJ. The effect of knee ankle foot orthosis in the treatment of Duchenne muscular dystrophy; review of the literature clinical rehab, 2000 April: (1), 14 (4): p. 343-59.
- Cervellati S, Bettini N, Moscato M, Gusella A, dema E, Maresi R. Surgical treatment of spinal deformities in Duchenne muscular dystrophy; A long-term following study. Eur spine J, 2004;13 (5):441-8.
- Darry C, Vivo DE, Salvatore D. Herditary and Acquired types of myopathy; Julia AM, Ralph DF, Catherine DD, Douglas JJ. Oski's Pediatrics, Principles and Practice, Philadelphia, PA, USA, Lippincott willams and Wilkins, 2006.
- Eckersley, PM. Elements of Pediatric Physiotherapy, Edinburgh, UK, Churchill Livingstone, 1993;187-202
- Elizabeth KE. Fundamentals of pediatrics'; Neuromuscular disorders, Paras Medical Publisher, 2002, p. 396-400.
- Finder JD, Birnkrant D, Carl J, et.al. Repiratory care of the patient with duchenne muscular dystrophy, ATS Consensus statement. Am J Respir Crit Care Med; 2004;170(4): 456-65.
- Hervey B, Sarnet. Neuromsuclar Disorders. Muscular Dystrophy; Behrman, Keliegman, Jenson. Nelson Textbook of Pediatrics, 7th Ed, Elsevier, Philadelphia, 2004; 2060-69.
- Jone HR, Dvivo DC, Darras DT. Neuromuscular disorders of infancy, childhood and adolescence, Bostan, Butterworth-Heinemann, 2003.
- Kent GA, Fred A, Ziter MF. Loss of strength and functional decline in Duchenne dystrophy. Arch Neuro; 1981; 38(7): 406-11.
- Pandya S, Julaine MF, Wendy MK, Jenny DR, Mindy O, Michael AP. Reliability of goniometric measurements in patients with Duchenne Muscular dystrophy, Phys ther, Sept 1985; vol 65 ( no. 9): 1339-42.
- Paul J, Vignos JR, Marilyn B, Wagner MA, et al. Evaluation of a program

for long-term treatment of Duchenne muscular dystrophy, Experience at the University Hospitals of Cleveland. The J Bone and Joint Surg, 78; 1844-52.

- Quinlivan R, Roper H, Davie M, Shaw NJ, Mc Donagh J, Bushby K - Report of a muscular dystrophy campaign funded workshop Brimingham, UK, Jan 16 th , 2004, Osteoporesis in Duchenne muscular dystrophy; its prevalence treatment and prevention. Neuromuscul Disord 2005;15(1):72-9.

- Ranbeck J, werge B, Madesen A, Marquardt J, Steffensen BF, Jeppesen J. Adult life with Duchenne muscular dystrophy; Observations among an emerging and unforeseen patient population, Pediatric Rehabil 2005;8(1):1-12.

- Richard ML, Neil CP, Robert JB. The Muscular Dystrophies: From Genes to Therapies, Phys Ther, 12, Dec, 2005; vol: 85 (no): 1372-88.

- Roz D, Anne K, Doreen D, Marina M, Lesley W. Duchenne muscular dystrophy Scottish physiotherapy management profile , April 2007.

- Stokes M. Physical management in Neurological Rehabilitation, Edinburgh, 2004; 347-66.

- Veena A, Agrawal, Sharma JP, et al. Anaesthetic Management of patient with Duchenne muscular dystrophy for orthopedic surgery. J Anaesth Clin Pharmacol,  2007;23(2); 201-02.

# Chapter

## 6

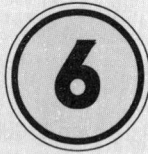

# Physical Therapy in Parkinson's Disease

## PARKINSON'S DISEASE (PD)

- Parkinson's disease was first described by James Parkinson in 1817. Parkinson disease (PD) is a progressive disease associated with a degeneration's of the dopamine producing cells in the substantia nigra (Brusse KJ, et al. 2005). It is the second most common cause of chronic neurological disability.
- People with Parkinson's disease are known to have a shuffling gait, difficulty initiating movements, a stooped forward posture, marked postural instability, bradykinetic movements, masked facial expression and tremor.

### Incidence

- The incidence of PD is 18 per 100000 of population per year, amounting to approximately 10000 new cases per year in the UK. (Jones D and Playfer J 2004).
- PD is more likely to occur in males, because females survive longer there is a fairly even distrubution of overall cases between the sexes.
- Affects 0.3% of total population (1% of population older than 55 years).

### Etiology

- Aging is not cause of parkinson's disease
- Toxin exposure
- Genetic predisposition and oxidative stress.

### Pathophysiology

- Dopamine depletion due to degeneration of the dopaminergic nigrostriatal system leads to an imbalance of dopamine and acetylcholine, which are neurotransmitters normally present in the corpus striatum.

### Clinical Manifestations

*Cardinal Features*

- Resting tremor

**Physical Therapy in Parkinson's Disease**

- Rigidity
- Bradykinesia
- Postural instability.

### Resting Tremor

- It is most common presenting feature
- Resting tremor of 4 to 6 cycles per second is most conspicuous at rest
- Although it may ultimately be present in all limbs.

### Rigidity

- Rigidity is an increase resistance to passive movement
- Parkinson's rigidity is characterized by an increased resistance to passive movement through out the entire range of motion, in both agonist and antagoinst muscle power
- Functional outcomes: Flexed posture, lack of trunk rotation, reduced joint range of movement during postural transitions and gait.

### Bradykinesia

- Bradykinesia is most commonly defined as slowness of voluntary movement. But it is also associated with slow and weak postural responses to perturbations and anticipatory postural adjustments.

### Postural Instability

- It is a common and serious problem in parkinson's disease. Up to 90% of all parkinson's patient to diminished in postural reactions
- Thirty eight of hundred patients with PD fall 13% experience fractures, 18% hospitatalization and 3% are confined wheelchair.

### Other Signs and Symptoms

- Immobile facial expression
- Infrequent blinking
- Myerson's sign (repetitive tapping over the bridge of the nose produces a sustained blink response)

- Impairment of swallowing
- Impairment of fine or rapidly alternating movements and micrographia
- Shuffling gait
- Unsteadiness on turning
- Difficult in stopping and a tendency to fall
- Sleep distrubance
- Urinary dysfunction
- Visual disturbances.

## Psychiatric Symptoms

- Depression and dementia

## Diagnosis

- Clinical Examination: It is based on presence of bradykinesia, muscular rigidity, resting tremor, and postural instability
- Magnetic Resonance Imaging (MRI) scans: Are normal, with variable amounts of atrophy
- Single photon emission computed tomography (SPECT): May shows decrease in dopamine transporters
- Positron emission tomography (PET): May show decreased tracer uptake in putamen.

# CLASSIFICATION OF DISABILITY

## Modified Hoehn and Yahr Score (1967) (Table 6.1)

| Table: 6.1: Modified Hoehn and Yahr score (1967) | |
|---|---|
| Stage | Description |
| 0 | No signs of disease |
| 1 | Unilateral disease |
| 1.5 | Unilateral plus axial movement |
| 2 | Bilateral disease, without impairment of balance |
| 2.5 | Mild bilateral disease; recovery on pull test |
| 3 | Mild to moderate bilateral disease; some postural instability; capacity for living independence |
| 4 | Severe disability; still able to walk or stand unassisted. |
| 5 | Wheelchair bound or bedridden unless aided. |

Physical Therapy in Parkinson's Disease

## ASSESSMENT

- Patient History
- Assess cognitive and behavioral status:
  - Intelectual impairment
  - Dementia
  - Check for memory status deficits
  - Bradphrenia (Slowing of thought processes)
  - Depression
- Assess communication:
  - Dysarthria
  - Hypophonia are common
  - Mask-like face with frequent blinking and expression, writing becomes slow
- Assess for oromotor and nutritional status:
  - Dysphagia is common problem (Chewing and swallowing).
- Assess respiratory status:
  - Breathing pattern, vital capacity, decreased chest expansion.
- Assess vision:
  - Check for blurring, cog wheeling eye pursuit
  - Decreased pupillary reflexes
- Assess skin integrity:
  - Edema may be occur in lower extrmities.
  - Increase sweating
  - Pressure sores in later stages
- Assess Muscle tone:
  - Check for rigidity including location, distrubution and symmetry between two sides of body, type (Cog-wheel, or lead-pipe)
- Assess ROM
  - Active range of motion (AROM), deformity associated with disuse and inactivity.
  - Contractures common in flexors, adductors.
  - Persistent posturing in kyphosis with forward posture
  - Many patients osteoporotic with high risk of fractures
- Assess muscle strngth
  - Weakness is associated with disuse atrophy
  - Assess torque output at varying speeds (Isokinetics)

- Assess motor control:
  - Assess for bradykinesia
  - Ability to inititate movement (number of freezing episodes, precipitating factors)
  - Assess reaction time versus movement time, overall poverty of movement
- Assess involuntary movements:
  - Check for presence of location of resting tremor.
  - Pill-rolling of hands
  - Postural tremors
- Assess for sensory and percept ual deficits:
  - Abnormal sensations (cramplike sensations, poorly localized).
  - Problems in spatial organization
  - Perception of vertical, extreme restlessness (akathisia)
- Assess balance
  *Berg Balance Scale*
  - Check for both static and dyanmic balance
  - Impaired postural reactions are common (worse with severity rigidity of trunk, lack of trunk rotation)
- Assess Gait:
  - Abnormal, involuntary in the speed of walking
  - Patient is to walk a fixed distance and recording the number of steps and the time taken to cover the distance
  - Assess for quality of the heel strike should be noted: Heel-toe, flat footed, toe-heel
  - Patient's ambulatory posture should be noted
- Assess functional abilities:
  - Turning over in bed
  - Sitting from lying
  - Standing from the sitting position
- Assess overall level of endurance:
  - 6 minte walk test
- Standard tests and measures in PD.

## Physical Therapy Intervention

- The aim of Physical therapy is to promote strength, increase flexibility, reeducate balance, to improve transfer activities, to training for joint mobility, improve gait and physical capacity in patients with Parkinson's disease ( Samrya HJ et al. 2006).

- Patients with Parkinson's disease (PD) face mounting mobility deficits, including with difficulties with transfers, posture, balance and walking. This frequency leads to loss of functional independence, fear of falls, injuries and inactivity, result in social isolation and an increased risk of osteoporesis or cardiovascular disease. Consequently, costs increase, and quality of life decreases. These mobility deficits are difficult to treat with drugs or neurosurgery
- Physical therapy is often prescribed next to medical treatment
- Six core areas for Physical therapy in PD were identified:
  1. Transfers ( e.g.) Turning in bed or raising from a chair)
  2. Posture (Including Neck and back Problems)
  3. Reaching and grasping
  4. Balance and falls (including fear of falls)
  5. Gait or walking
  6. Physical capacity and activity.

## Recommendations of Physical Therapy Intervention

I. Application of cueing strategies to improve gait
II. Application of cognitive movement strategies to improve transfers
III. Specific exercises to improve balance
IV. Training of joint mobility and muscle power to improve physcial capacity.

## Cueing Strategies

- In Patient with Parkinson's disease, gait is improved by applying visual or auditory cues, which have trained during active gait training
- Cues are stimuli from environment or generated by the patient, which the patient uses, consciously or not , to facilitate (automatic or repetitive) movements. It is not clear exactly how cues improve movement
- Perhaps they provide external rhythm that can compensate for the improperly supplied internal rhythm of the basal ganglia,

correct motor set deficiency or ( in cases of visual cues ) generate optical flow that activates cerebellar visual-motor pathway. Not all patients benefit equally from using cues

- Cues can be divided into four groups :
  - Auditory cues ( e.g.) the use of walkman with rhythmic music, a metraonome or counting (by the patient, partner, or caretaker)
  - Visual cues (e.g. stepping over stripes on the floor or over the grip of an inverted walking stick, or focusing on an object (e.g. a clock) in the environment
  - Tactile cues (e.g. tapping on the hip or the leg)
  - Cognitive cues (e.g. a mental image of the appropriate step length).

## Cognitive Movement Strategies

- Cognitive movement strategies to improve performance of transfers
- In this strategies, automated movements are transformed into a series of submovements that have to be executed in a fixed order
- The course of the movement is there by reorganized in such a way that the activity can be performed consciously

## Balance

- Balance training (where patients are taught to use visual and vestibular feedback)
- Combined with lower extremity strength training is effective in improving balance in patients with PD.

## Physical Activity

- The exercise program aim is to improve range of motion combined with activity related to (e.g. gait or balance exercise)
- Improves ADL functioning
- Strength training program increasing muscle power ( strengthen low back and hip extensors)
- Range of motion trunk exercises

- Use mirrors to correct posture
  - Teach Relaxation skills
  - Improve cardiovascular endurance
  - Teach energy conservation techniques
  - Speech and breathing exercises
  - Home health aides in assisting patient (appropriate aids and adaptive equipment).

## BIBLIOGRAPHY

- Bergen JL, Toole T, Elliot RG, Wallace B, Robinson K, Maitland CG. Aerobic exercise intervention improves aerobic capacity and Movement initiation in Parkinson's disease patients. Neuro Rehab, 2002; 17:161-8.
- Bridgewater KJ, Sharpe M - Trunk muscle training and early parkinson disease. Phys Ther; 1997; vol 13: 139-53.
- Brusse KJ, Zimdars S, Zaleski KR, Steffen TM. Testing Functional performance in people with Parkinson's disease. Phys Ther, 2005; vol 85(2): 134-41.
- Comella CL, Stebbins Gt, Brown TN, Goetz CG. Physical therapy and Parkinson's disease; A Controlled Clinical trial. Neurology, 1994; 44(1); 376-78.
- Cynthia L, Comelia, Glenn T, Stebbins, Nancy BT, Christopher GG. Physicaltherapy and Parkinson disease, neurology, Am Acad of Neuro; 1994.
- Formisano R, Pratesi L, Modarelli FL, Bontifati V, Meco G. Rehabilitation and Parkinson's disease, scand J Rehabil Med, 1992;24:157-60.
- Janice JE. Stepping forward gait rehabilitation; phys Ther, 2010; 90(2): 146-8.
- Jobges M, Heuschkel, Pretzel C, Illhardt C, Renner, Hummelsheim H. Repetitive training of componensatory steps; a therapeutic approach for Postural instability in Parkinson disease. J Neurol Neuro surg Psychiatry, 2004;75:1682-7.
- Keus SH, Munnekke M, Nijkrake MJ, Kwakkel G, Bloem BR. Physical therapy in Parkinson's Disease: Evaluation and future challenges. Mov Disord, 2009;24(1): p. 1-14.
- Laurie AK, Fay BH. Delaying mobility in people with Parkinson's disease using a sensorimotor agility exercise program. Phys Ther, 2009; 89(4): 384-93.
- Meg EM, Clarissa LM, Margaret LS. Jacquelin Perry Special Issue; Stepping forward with gait rehabilitation: Striding out with Parkinson's disease: Evidence Based Physical therapy for gait disorders; Phys Ther; 2010, 90 (2), p. 280-8.

- Morris ME. Movement disorders in people with Parkinson disease: A model for Physical therapy. Phys Ther, 2000; 80(6): 578-97.
- Protas EJ, Mitchell K, Willams A, Qureshy H, Carollne KL. Gait and Step training to reduce falls in Parkinson's disease. Neuro rehab; 1993.
- Samrya HT, Keus, Bastiaan RB, Krik jM, et al. Evidence base analysis of Physical therapy in Parkinson disease with recommendations for practice and research. Mov Dis, 2006; 22(4): 451-60.
- Schenkan ML, Clark K, Xie T, Kuchibhata M, et al. Spinal movement and Performance of a standing reach, Task in participants with and without Parkinson's disease. Phys Ther; 2001; 81 (8): p. 1400- 1

# Chapter

//////////////////////////

## (7)

# Spinal Cord Injury Rehabilitation

## SPINAL CORD INJURY (SCI)

- Spinal cord injury (SCI), whether of traumatic or nontraumatic etiology, often results in significant and catastrophic dysfunction and disability. It physically and psychologically affects not only the individual but also the family and society. Early rehabilitation in an organized multidisciplinary SCI care system has been shown to be beneficial, with lower mortality, decreased pressure sores, slightly greater chance of neurologic recovery, and shorter lengths of stay with lower hospital charges.

### Incidence

- An annual incidence of 15 to 40 traumatic SCI cases per million populations has been reported worldwide, and a conservative estimate for India would be 20,000 cases are added every year
- Sixty to seventy percent of them are illiterate, poor villagers
- In Asia pacific region, Australia with 2003 population of 20 million reported an incidence of 300-400 new cases per year or 15 to 20 per million, and a prevalence of 10,000 persons with Spinal cord injury.

### Common Causes of SCI

- Industrial injuries 34.5%
- Road traffic accidents 33.1%
- Cervical injuries 44%
- Thoraco lumbar injuries 26.6%
- Lumbar injuries 20.8%.

### Mode of Injury

- The most common cause of injury was fall from height including roof, trees, electricity pole, and motor vehicle accidents
- Falls were more prominent in second and third decades. Road side accidents were commoner in third and fourth decade.

### Spinal Cord Syndromes

- Brown-Sequard syndrome

- Central cord syndrome
- Anterior cord syndrome
- Conus medullaris syndrome
- Cauda eqina syndrome.

## Brown-Sequard Syndrome

- Hemisection of spinal cord due to trauma, tumor
- Ipsilateral paralysis and loss of proprioception due to the crossing of the corticospinal tracts and dorsal columns in the brainstem
- Produces contralateral loss of pain and temperature sensation due to local crossing of spinothalamic tracts in the spinal cord.

## Anterior Cord Syndrome

- Damage is in anterior cord resulting in loss of motor function and pain and temperature with preservation of light touch, proprioception and position sense.

## Central Cord Syndrome

- A lesion in the central gray matter and medial white matter tracts in the cervical spinal cord due to compression /ischemia
- Usually seen in hyperextension injuries to the cervical spine, particularly in older persons with degenerative arthritis in the cervical spine
- Greater weakness in upper extremities than lower extremities with sacral sparing.

## Cauda Equina Syndrome

- Lesion of the lumbosacral nerve roots within the neural canal because lesion involves the peripheral nerves
- Results in flaccid paralysis and sensory loss to the lower extremities
- Lower motor neurone, autonomous or nonreflex bladder.

## Sacral Sparing

- Sparing of tracts to sacral segments, with preservation of perianal sensation, rectal sphincter tone and active toe flexion.

## CLASSIFICATION (FIGS 7.1 AND 7.2 )

### Tetraplegia (Quadriplegia)

- Impairment or loss of motor, sensory and or autonomic function in cervical segments of the spinal cord
- Injury occurs between C1 and C8 involves all four extremities and trunk.

### Paraplegia

- Impairment or loss of motor, sensory and or autonomic function in thoracic, lumbar or sacral segments of the spinal cord
- Injury occurs between T1 and T12, involves both lower extremities and trunk.

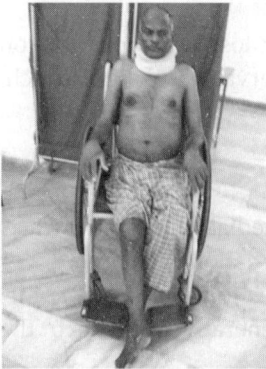

Fig. 7.1: Paraplegia

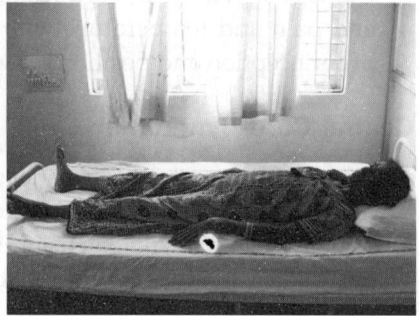

Fig. 7.2: Quadriplegia

## American Spinal injury Association (ASIA) Impairment Scale (Mcdonald JW and Sadowsky C, 2002)

- **A = complete:** No motor or sensory function is preserved in the sacral segments S4-S5
- **B = Incomplete:** Sensory but not motor function is preserved below the neurological level and includes the sacral segments S4-S5
- **C = Incomplete:** Motor function is preserved below the neurological level, and more than half of key muscles below the neurological level have a muscle grade than 3

- **D = Incomplete:** Motor function is preserved below the neurological level, and at least half of key muscles below the neurological level have a muscle grade of 3 (or) more.

## MEDICAL COMPLICATIONS OF SPINAL CORD INJURY

### Deep vein Thrombosis (DVT): see Chapter (4)

*Autonomic Dysreflexia (AD)*

- Autonomic dysreflexia is an acute syndrome of uninhibited sympathetic discharge as a result of noxious stimuli
- This condition can occur in any patient with spinal injury at level of above T5
- Symptoms: Paroxysmal hypertension (20-40 mm Hg increase above base line)–especially in tetraplegia, other signs/symptoms include headache, bradycardia/tachycardia, flushing and sweating
- Treatment: The first and most important goal is to decrease blood pressure, sit the patient upright and remove support hose/abdominal binder. Remove tight clothing and check the skin
  - Therapist should monitor symptoms
  - The patient should be positioned in sitting immediately to create postural hypotension or decrease the blood pressure
  - This can be performed only if the patient's spine is stable enough for him/her to be sitting position
  - Therapist should check the catheter and tubing, empty the leg bag, if it is full and depending upon the severity of the symptoms.

### Heterotopic Ossification

- Heterotopic ossification is defined as the formation of new osseous material in tissues where bone formation does not usually occur
- Ossification of soft tissues near and around joint regions occurs most commonly after spinal cord injury, traumatic injuries, burns, general trauma, total joint surgeries and occasionally in pediatric amputation patients

- SCI incidence of 15-40 %, with severe functional impairment in 18-12%
- Increased incidence if SCI is complete, secondary trauma, and associated with tetraplegia
- Typically, the hip, knee, elbow, and shoulder joints are most frequently involved
- Specific causes are unknown
- Symptoms: Loss of range motion(ROM), stiffness in affected area, pain , swelling, heat, and warmth
- Physical Therapy treatment:
  - Positioning
  - Gentle active–assisted ROM exercises, especially during acute stage of inflammation; they generally help to prevent ankylosis and promote better overall function
- Stretching exercises.

## Pressure sores (Decubitus Ulcers)

- Pressure sores can result from any prolonged, unchanged position
- Ulcers are found most frequently over bony prominences exposed to compressing surfaces.
- Incidence among patients with spinal cord injury (SCI) ranges from 24 to 59%
- Prevention:
  - Relief of pressure, water bed or airfilled cushion or mattress/ air fluidized beds
  - Patient should be repositioned every two hours
  - Assess skin with each turning.

## Bladder/ Bowel Problems

- Bladder and bowel can be a primary disabling problem for patients with spinal cord injury
- Urination is controlled by the conus medullaris, and primary reflex control is in the sacral segments
- Spinal shock and lesions above conus medullaris result in the bladder being flaccid, absent reflexes, a reflex neurogenic bladder and reflex bowel

- Lesions of conus medullaris result in the bladder being non-reflexive, decreased tone of the ureteral sphincter and perineal muscles and nonreflex bowel.

## Spasticity

- Spasticity secondary to SCI and other CNC injury damage is common
- Spasticity developed in 67% of SCI patients by discharge (of first injury-related hospitalization (Timothy LS, 2009)
- It is more prevalent in cervical and high thoracic injuries than in lower thoracic or Lumbosacral injuries
- Clinical manifestations of hypertonicity (increased muscle tone), clonus (a series of rapid muscle contractions), spastic paralysis, hyperreflexia (exaggerated deep tendon reflexes), Babinski's sign and clasp-knife rigidity
- Assessment: On Physical examination, spasticity can be assessed using the Ashworth scales (original and modified), spasm scale (Table 7.2), and physicians rating scale
- The Ashworth scale (or modified Ashworth scale) measuring rigidity on a 1-5 basis and the spasm scale, quantifying number of spasms per hour (Table 7.1).

| Table 7.1: Ashworth and Spasm scale | |
|---|---|
| Score | Degree of muscle tone |

### ASHWORTH SCALE

| | |
|---|---|
| 1 | No increase in tone |
| 2 | Slight increase in tone , giving a "catch" when affected part moved in flexion or Extension. |
| 3 | More marked increase in tone, but affected part easily flexed. |
| 4 | Considerable increase in tone; passive movement difficult. |
| 5 | Affected part rigid in flexion or extension |

### MODIFIED ASHWORTH SCALE

| | |
|---|---|
| 0 | No increase in tone |
| 1 | Slight increase in muscle tone, manifested by a catch and release or minimal resistance at the end of the ROM when the affected part(s) is moved in flexion or extension |

*Contd...*

| | |
|---|---|
| 1+ | Slight increase in muscle tone, manifested by a catch, followed by minimal resistance<br>Throughout remainder (less than half) of the ROM |
| 2 | More marked increase in muscle tone through most of the ROM, but affected parts easily moved |
| 3 | Considerable increase in muscle tone; passive movement difficult |
| 4 | Affected parts rigid in flexion or extension. |

### Table 7.2: Spasm Scale

| Score | Criteria |
|-------|----------|
| 0 | None |
| 1 | No spontaneous spasms, vigorous sensory and motor stimulation results in spasms |
| 2 | Occasional spontaneous and easily induced spasms |
| 3 | More than 1 but < 10 spontaneous spasms per hour |
| 4 | > 10 spontaneous spasms per hour. |

## Treatment

- The best management is prevention in the first few months after injury ( Bernes et al, 2001)
- Physical therapy is usually necessary in every spastic patient while, proper positioning, orthotics, splints, regular stretching exercises, aquatic therapy, biofeedback, cryotherapy
- The medical approach is through pharmacology, the drugs (commonly used baclofen, dantrolene and tizanidine) is universally effective or indeed predictable in its effect (Paddison, S, Middleton F, 2004)
- Use of intramuscular botulinum toxin, phenol nerve block
- Surgery: Tendon relase and nerve divisions, e.g. obturator neurectomy.

## ASSESSMENT

### Respiratory System

- Assess for Oxygen saturation level
- All respiratory muscles, abdominal muscles
- Auscultation
- Coughing.

## Cardiovascular System

- Pulse
- Blood pressure
- Heart sounds.

## Gastrointestinal Tract

- Abdomen, bowel sounds normal/abnormal.

## Urinary Tract

- Voluntary bladder control
- Indwelling catheter was inserted on admission.

## Sensory Examination

*Examination for Sensations Tests was Performed*

- Touch, pain, joint position, deep pressure
- Record level of normal sensation by drawing a line on the patients skin.

## Motor Examination

- The Royal Medical Research Council of Great Britain scale can be based to assess power (Table 7.2)
- Abdominal and erector spinae muscle group could not be tested according to this scale and only a subjective grading based on palpation was done

| Table 7.3: Royal Medical Research Council of Great Britiain Strength grading scale | |
|---|---|
| *Grade* | *Strength* |
| 0 | No contraction |
| 1 | Flicker or Trace of contraction |
| 2 | Active movement with gravity eliminated |
| 3 | Active movement against activity |
| 4 | Active movement against resistance |
| | 4- Slight resistance |
| | 4 Moderate resistance |
| | 4+ Strong resistance |
| 5 | Normal strength. |

| Table 7.4: Frankel Scale | |
|---|---|
| Grade | Description |
| A or 1 | Complete motor and sensory paralysis below the lesion. |
| B or 2 | Complete motor and sensory paralysis, but some residual sensory<br>Perception below the lesion. |
| C or 3 | Residual motor function, but of no practical use. |
| D or 4 | Useful subnormal motor function below the lesion. |
| E or 5 | Normal. |

## REFLEXES

- Deep tendon reflexes (DTR): Biceps, triceps, patellar, ankle jerk.
- Superficial reflexes: Abdominal (Upper, Lower) reflex, cremasteric, bublocavernous reflex.
- Grading: 0- 4

## Investigations

### Plain X-rays

- Cervical spine X-ray: from craniocervical junction to C7/T1 junction. Anterior posterior, lateral, oblique or swimmer view may be necessary to demonstrate lower cervical vertebrae.
- Thoracolumbar spine X-ray: Anterior posterior and lateral view to rule out a second injury or demonstrate fractures in case of suspected thoracolumbar injury.

*CT scan and MRI Scan.* Of the fractured segment may demonstrate cord involument or spinal canal obstruction.

*CT Myelography.* May demonstrate spinal block, although MRI has largely replace it.

*Spinal Angiography.* May demonstrate vascular involument especially in patient with SCI

## Acute Physical therapy Management of Spinal cord injury

**Goal:** Purpose of rehabilitation after spinal cord injury (SCI), to help the patient TO establish control over his/her own health and life.

Spinal Cord Injury Rehabilitation

**Aspects of Rehabilitation include:**

- Psychological support
- Clear ventilation
- Improve chest expansion
- Skin care
- Prevent pressure sores
- Prevent contractures or stiffness.
- Regaining as muscle strength and function in the trunk and extremities as possible.
- Independent personal and community mobility.
- Management of bladder and bowel function
- Psychosocial and sexual function
- Independent living and vocational rehabilitation.

## Respiratory Care in Tetraplegia

- Patients with lesions of T1 and above lose some 40-50% of their respiratory function but most patients with cervical injuries have an initial vital capacity of only 1.5 Liters or less
- Teach breathing exercise to encourage chest expansion and improve ventilation
- Incentive spirometry is useful for mid thoracic lesions and above.
- Assisted cough
- Postural drainage
- Inspiratory muscle training devices are of great benefit for improving forced vital capacity (FVC ) (Houch, 2001).

## Physical Therapy Intervention of Paraplegia

- Motivation and self confidence are also major factors in successful rehabilitation. They are required, first to accept irreversible facts
- Physical therapy is usually a major part of the treatment program in spinal cord injury
- Interventions for SCI patients includes:
  - Positioning: To prevent deformity and damage to skin, joints, or soft tissues. Prevention compression of veins, especially in the calf region.
  - Special beds, e.g. water bed or air cushion matteress bed.

- Frequently turning the patient's position: Supine to side lying, rotation right and left lying at 2 hours once
- Skin must be inspected to detect to any signs of pressure sores
- Chest physical therapy helps to clear lungs secretion (percussion, shaking, vibration techniques)
- Deep breathing exercise
- Coughing techniques
- Passive ROM exercise: Maintains ROM, and improves blood circulation
- Progressive resistance exercise: These are exercises done with weights, pulleys, and special exercise machines
- Independent passive movements
- Mat class: Working on a mat, the patient relearns and practices the skills needed for independent living; changing position in bed getting and moving from one place to another.
- Rolling on side
- Sitting up from lying on back and prone
- Balance in long and high sit
- Lifting arm, rhythmic stabilization techniques, moving in out of the position, throwing ball
- Transfer training in high sit and long sit
- Tilt Table: A table that can be positioned at various angles to the horizontal helps the cardiovascular system read just to upright position after has been in bed for extended periods.
- Walking Rehabilitation: Standing in the tilt table to standing between the parallel bars
- Standing balance, swing through gait training and elbow crutches.

## Occupational Therapy

- Transfer to the bed and the toilet
- Endurance training by pushing his/her wheelchair
- Basic wheelchair manipulation
- Balance in sitting
- Handling in wheelchair
- Back wheel balance
- Education.

Spinal Cord Injury Rehabilitation

## Spinal Orthosis

### Cervical Orthosis

- **Aim:** Control pain, protect further injury, limit or restrict movement, support soft tissues, control cervical spine position.

### Sterno-Occupital-Mandibular Immobilization (SOMI)

- Acronym for sternal occipital mandibular immobilization
- Good for bracing against flexion, allows patient to eat without mandibular support (Shehu, BB, 2004).
- A method of external stabilization for the cervical vertebrae.

### Thoracic-Lumbar- Sacral Orthosis (TLSO)

- TLSO used depends on stability of fracture site and ligamentous involument
- Three point force control system with anterior compression of abdomen
- Stabilize or correct thorcolumbar sacral spine alignment
- Protect structures.

### Weiss Springs

- An internal stabilization method for the thoracic and lumbar vertebrae.

## Common Splints Used in Tetraplegia

### C7- L1 injury

- Hip guidance orthosis (HGO)
- Reciprocal gait orthosis.

### T6-T12 Level

- Caliper walker with rollator and crutches.

### L3 level

- Appropriate orthosis or walking aid

- Ankle -Foot-Drop splint (AFO)
- Hip-Knee-Ankle Foot orthosis (HKAFO)
- Knee-Ankle-Foot orthosis (KAFO).

### Ambulatory Aids

- Canadian type of elbow crutches
- Walking frames
- Wheelchair.

## ACTIVE ASSISTED FACILITATION OF MOVEMENT TECHNIQUES FOR PARAPLEGIA

### Functional Electrical Stimulation (FES)

- FES used to improve hand function in tetraplegics
- Used for urinary /bowel dysfunction
- To improve cardiovascular function.

### Body Weight Support Treadmill Training (BWSTT)

- BWSTT gained impetus with reports of functional improvement after ambulation training on a treadmill
- BWSTT ambulation training wearing harness supports for 30 to 60 minutes, 5 days a week
- Significantly, after training, patients were able to walk 100-2000 m on a static surface despite absent voluntary activity in the paralyzed limb at rest.

### Robotic Devices

- Robotic device use of automated driven gait orthosis ambulation training has been proposed to significantly, reduce the load on therapists during ambulation training.

### Neural Activity Controlled Prosthesis

- Recent developments in the field of neural prosthesis include improvements in important area of brain machine interface (BMI).

Spinal Cord Injury Rehabilitation

## Pain Management

- Electrothermotherapy, positioning, TENS, movement re-education and acupuncture.

## BIBLIOGRAPHY

- American Spinal injury Association: International standards for neurological classification of spinal cord injury. Revised; Chicago; American Spinal injury Association, 2000.
- Brammmer CM, Catherine Spires, M. Manual of Physical medicine and rehabilitation. Elsevier, 2002; p. 119-38.
- Field Fote EC. Spinal cord control movement: Implications for locomotor rehabilitation following spinal cord Injury. Phys Ther, 2000; 80(5): 477-84.
- Gourassini MA, Noton JA, Ducherer JN, Roy FD, Yang JF. Changes in locomotor muscle activity after treadmill training in subjects with in complete spinal cord injury. J Neuro Physiol, 2009;101(2):969-79.
- Kathleen A, Curtis , Karry lMH. Spinal cord injury community follow up: Role of physical therapist; Phys Ther, 1986; 66(9): 1370-5.
- Katz RT, Spasticity, In: O' Young B, Young MA, steins SA. PM and R secrets, phildelphia; Hanley and Belfus, 1997; p 487.
- Mangold S, Keller T, Curt A, Diet V. Transcutaneous functional electrical stimulation for grasping in subjects with cervical spinal cord injury. Spinal cord, 2005;43: 1-13.
- National institute of Neurological Disorders and Stroke (National institute of Health) http//www.ninds.gov/disorders/spasticity/ spasticity/htm, accessed june 21, 2009.
- Pollack SF, Axen K, Spietholz N, Levin N, Haas F, Ragnarsson KT. Aerobic training effects of electrically induced lower extremity exercise in spinal cord injured people. Arch Phys Med Rehabili, 1969; 70;(3): 214-5.
- Peter Ac, Lim, Adela MT. Recovery and regeneration after spinal cord injury: A review and summery of recent literature. Ann Acad med Singapore, 2007; 36:49-57.
- Riva G, Italiano IA. Virtual reality in paraplegia; A test bed application. The International J. Virtual Reality, 2001; 5(1): 1-10.
- Shehu BB, Ismail NJ. Continuing education: Practical management of spinal cord injury, annals African medicine; 2004; 3(1): 46-52.

- Staas WE, Formal CS, Freedman MK, et al. Spinal cord injury and Spinal cord injury Medicine. In DeLisa JA (ed): Rehabilitation Medicine, Principles and Practice, 3rd ed, Philadelphia, Lippincott willams and wilkins, 1998, p. 1276-7.
- Timothy L, Sternberg. Treatment of Spasticity associated with spinal cord injury and other central nervous system damage. North East Flordia medicine, 2009; 60(3): p. 19-22.
- Wening A, Mullers S. Laufband. Locomotion with body weight support improved walking in persons with severe spinal cord injuries, Paraplegia, 1992; 30: 229-38.
- Yen HL, Chua K, Chan W. Spinal cord Injury rehabilitation in singapore. Int. J. Rehabili Res, 1998;21: 375-87.

# Chapter

////////////////////////////////

# 8

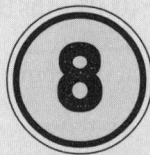

# Physical Therapy in Cerebral Palsy

## CEREBRAL PALSY (CP)

- The term cerebral palsy (CP) was first used by William Osler in 1887 but William Little in 1862 is credited with first describing and classifing the motor syndromes of CP.
- Cerebral palsy refers to a group of conditions characterized by abnormalities of movement and posture after nonprogressive lesions of the immature brain.

### Incidence

- The incidence of CP per 1000 births by birth weight is 90 among infants weight less than 1500 g
- Due to increased survival of premature infants with low birth weight.

### Etiology (Table 8.1)

- In 80% cases, features were identified pointing to antenatal factors causing abnormal brain development (Michael VJ 2008)
- Ten percent of children with CP had evidence of intrapartum asphyxia
- Intra uterine exposure to maternal infection (Chorioamnionitis, inflammation of placental membranes, umbilical cord inflammation, foul- smelling aminiotic fluid, maternal sepsis, temperature >38° during labor, urinary tract infection
- Low birth weight < 1000 g at birth
- Premature infants
- Intracerebral hemorrhage and periventricular leukomalacia (PVL).

| Table 8.1: Risk Factor | | |
|---|---|---|
| Prenatal | Perinatal | Postnatal |
| Congenital malformations | prematurity (<32 weeks) | Trauma |
| Socioeconomic factors | Birth weight , 2500 gm | Infection |
| Intrauterine infections | Growth retardation | Intracranial hemorrhage |

*Contd...*

*Contd...*

| Prenatal | Perinatal | Postnatal |
|---|---|---|
| Teratogenic mental retardation | Abnormal presentations | Coagulopathies |
| Maternal seizures | Trauma | |
| Maternal hyperthyroidism | Infection | |
| Placental complications | Bradycardia and hypoxia | |
| Additional trauma | Seizures | |
| Multiple gestation | Hyperbilirubinemia. | |

## Classification of Cerebral Palsy

- Spastic diplegia
- Spastic quadriplegia
- Hemiplegia
- Athetoid, Dyskinetic
- Mixed.

## CLINICAL MANIFESTATIONS

### Spastic Diplegic Cerebral Palsy (Little Disease)

- It is most common type of cerebral palsy (80% of cases)
- Lesions motor cortex
- Eighty percent cases are diplegic child

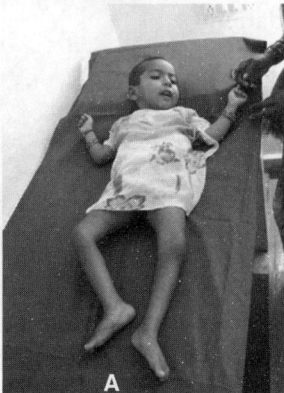

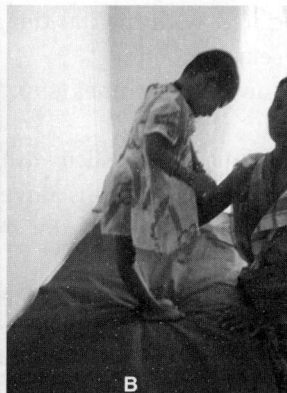

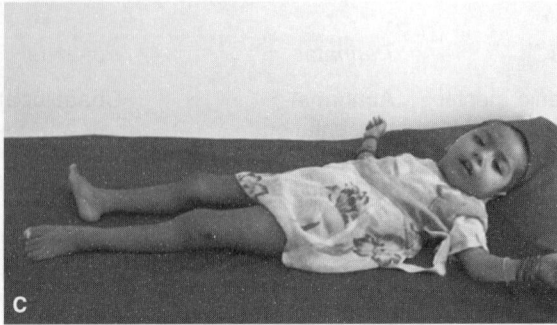

**Figs 8.1 A to C:** Spastic diplegic child

- Major causes: Prematurity, ischemia, infection, endocrine/ metabolic, e.g. thyroid
- Involves legs more than arms
- Delayed walking
- Scissoring posture
- Disuse atrophy and impaired growth of lower extremities
- Equino varus deformity
- Ankle clonus
- Bilateral Babinski sign is positive.

## Quadriplegia (Fig. 8.2)

- Quadriplegia is most severe form of CP because of marked motor impairment of all extremities and associated with mental retardation and seizures
- Swallowing difficulties (suprabulbar palsy)
- Hypertonia and spasticity to all limbs
- Decreased spontaneous movements
- Brisk reflexes and plantar extensor responses
- Flexion contractures of knees and elbows
- Speech and Visual impairments.

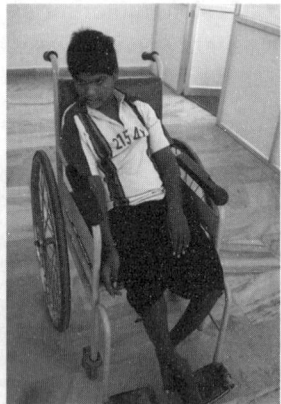

**Fig. 8.2:** Quadriplegic cerebral palsy

## Hemiplegia (Fig. 8.3)

- Paralysis or weakness of one side of the upper and lower extremity
- Arms is often more involved than the leg and difficulty in hand actitivities
- Walking is delayed until 18 to 24 months
- Circumductive gait
- Examination:
  - Spasticity is apparent in the affected extremities, particularly in ankle (Equino varus deformity of the foot).
- Increased tone
- Dystonic posture
- Deep tendon reflexes are increased
- Ankle clonus and a Babinski sign may be present.

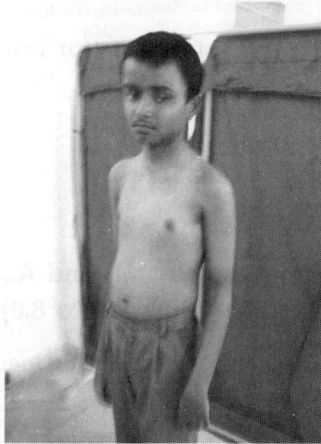

**Fig. 8.3:** Hemiplegic CP child

## Athetoid (Choreoathetoid or Extrapyramidal CP)

- Less common in spastic CP
- Hypotonic with poor head control and marked head lag
- Rigidity and dystonia
- Feeding may be difficult
- Tongue thrust and drooling may be prominent
- Speech problem (oropharyngeal muscle are involved).

### Diagnosis

**MRI Scan of Brain:** To determine location and extent of structural lesions or associated congenital malformations.

**CT Scan:** Useful for detecting calcifications associated with congenital infections.

## PHYSICAL THERAPY MANAGEMENT

### AIM

- Improve muscle strength
- Improve local muscular endurance
- Maintain or improve joint range of motion
- Decrease and prevent joint contractures
- Improve balance
- Postural control
- Mobility and ability to transfer (for instance from bed to wheelchair).
- Gait
- ADLs.

### Treatment /Techniques

### Passive range of motion (PROM) and Active range of motion (AROM) exercise (Figs 8.4 to 8.6)

- Repetitive PROM exercise to improve and maintain joint mobility.

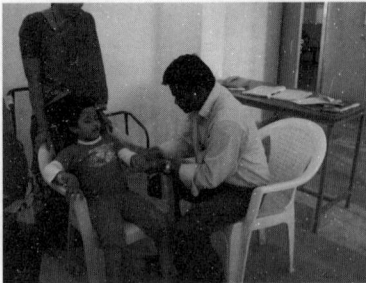

Fig. 8.4: PROM exercise with elbow flexion

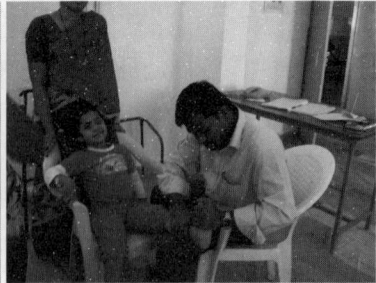

Fig. 8.5: PROM exercise in ankle dorsiflexion

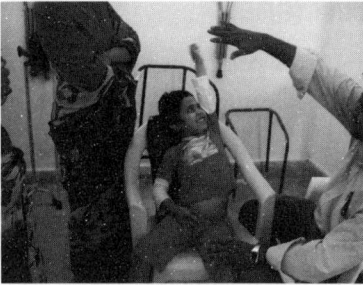

Fig. 8.6: AROM exercise in shoulder flexion

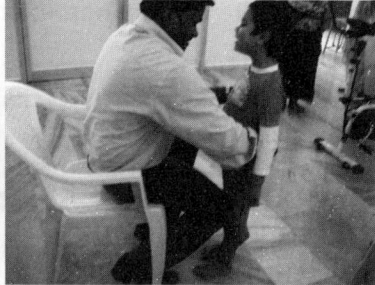

Fig. 8.7: Posture correction and weight bearing of the both lower extremity

## Passive, Static, Gentle Stretching (Figs 8.7 to 8.11)

• Are performed on individual joints to decrease and prevent joint contractures. Such stretches should be performed with in a pain free joint ROM.

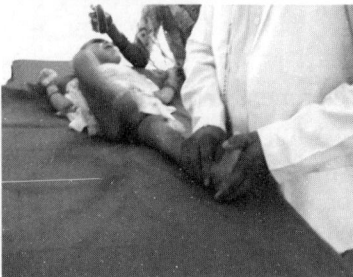

Fig. 8.8: Left side Calf muscle stretching

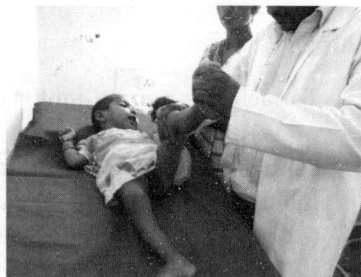

Fig. 8.9: Hamstrings stretching

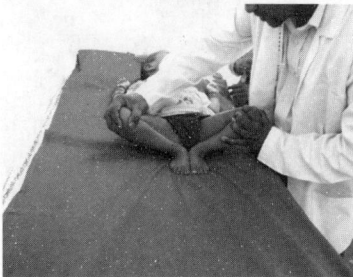

Fig. 8.10: Adductors muscles stretching

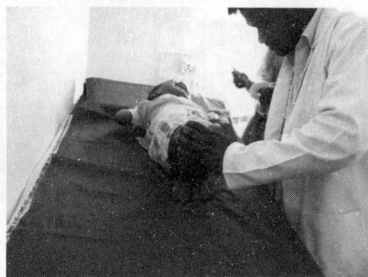

Fig. 8.11: Pelvic raising and TA stretch

### Progressive Resistance exercise (PRE)

- Used to improve muscle strength. A program that uses low resistance and more repetitions will enhance local muscular endurance.

### Neuro-Developmental Therapy (NDT)

- In 1940, Berta and Karl Bobath was first described therapeutic approach of Neuro-developmental therapy (NDT)
- It is most popular therapeutic approach interventions for the treatment of children with cerebral palsy.

### Basic Principle

- The motor abnormalities in children with cerebral palsy are due to failure of normal development of postural control and reflexes because of the underlying dysfunction of the central nervous system (Butler C, 2001).

### Aim

- To facilitate normal motor development and function and to prevent development of secondary impairments due to muscle contractions and joint and limb deformities
- Intensive NDT - 1 hour per day for 5 days per week and reported to be more effective (Patel DR, 2005).

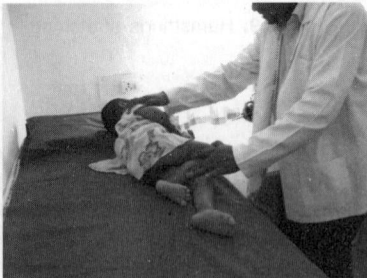

Fig. 8.12: Supine to side lying rolling mobility training

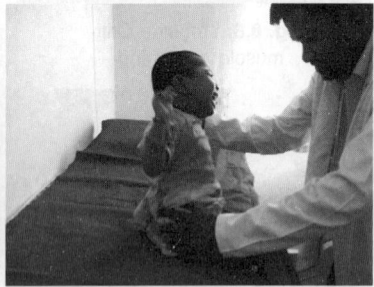

Fig. 8.13: Trunk control reeducation

Physical Therapy in Cerebral Palsy

## Sensory Integration (SI)

- The theory of sensory integration was originally developed by A. Jean Ayres in the 1970
- *Principle:* In developing treatment approaches for children with sensory processing difficulties, including CP
- The SI model was developed to treat learning difficulties
- The SI theory is to develop and execute a normal adaptive behavioral response, the child must be able to optimally receive, modulate, integrate, and process the sensory information
- Aim: To facilitate the normal development and improve the child's ability to process and integrate sensory information (visual, perceptual, proprioceptive, auditory, etc.)
- Improve functional capabilities in daily life activities. (Figs 8.12 to 8.18).

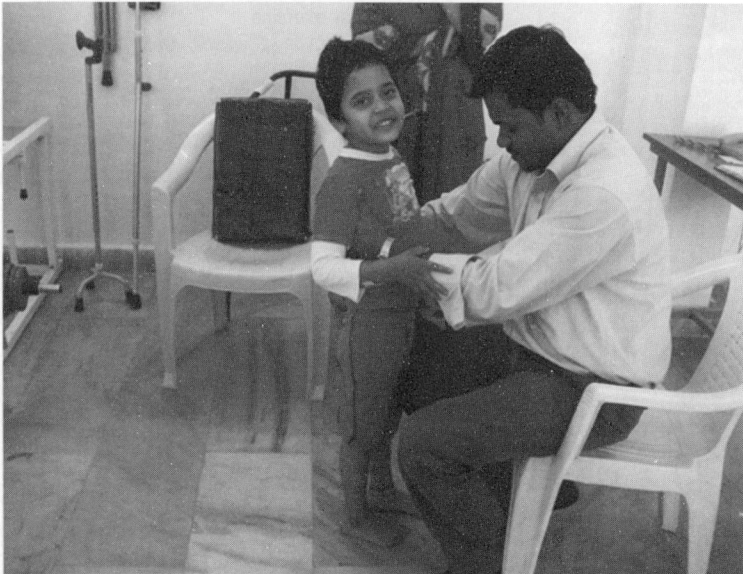

**Fig. 8.14:** Postural control re-training

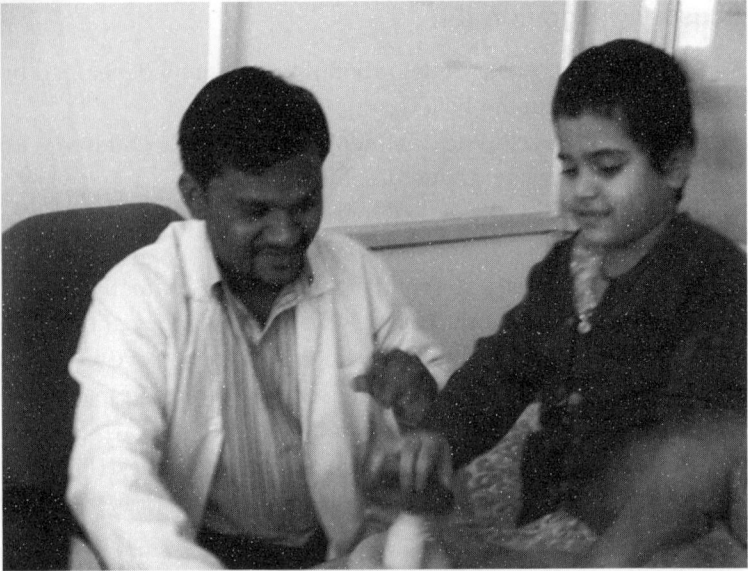

Fig. 8.15: Wrist exercise

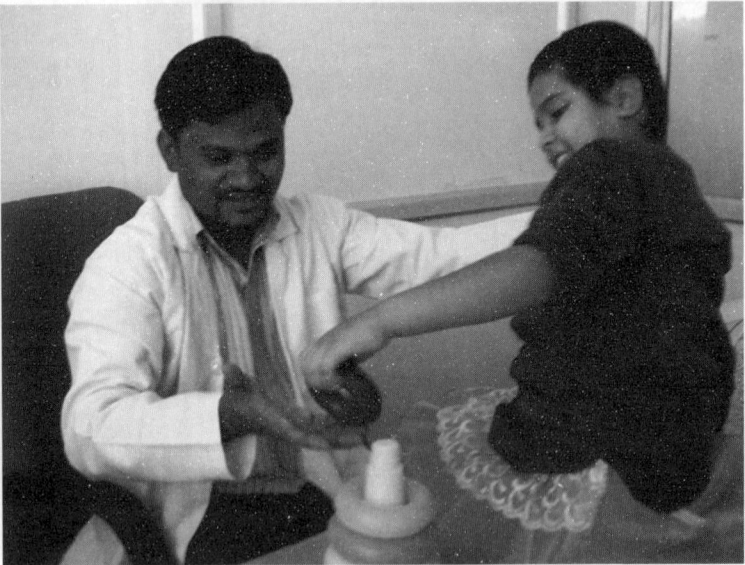

Fig. 8.16: ADLs training

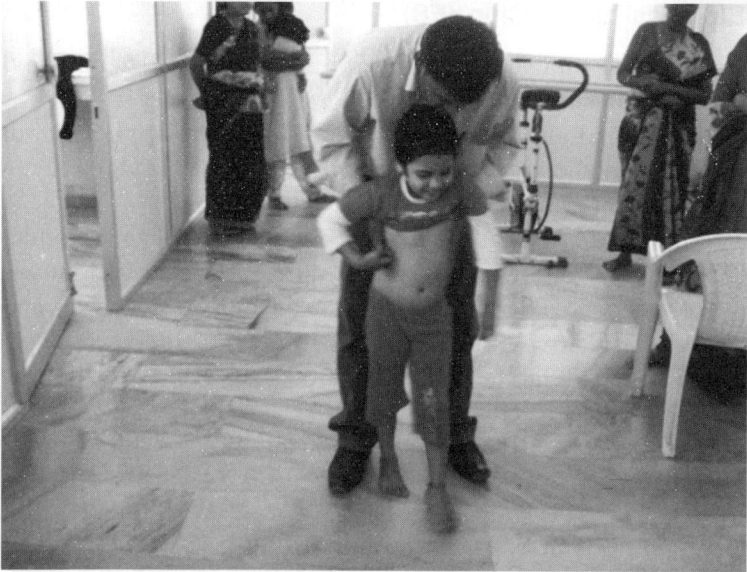

**Fig. 8.17:** Gait training

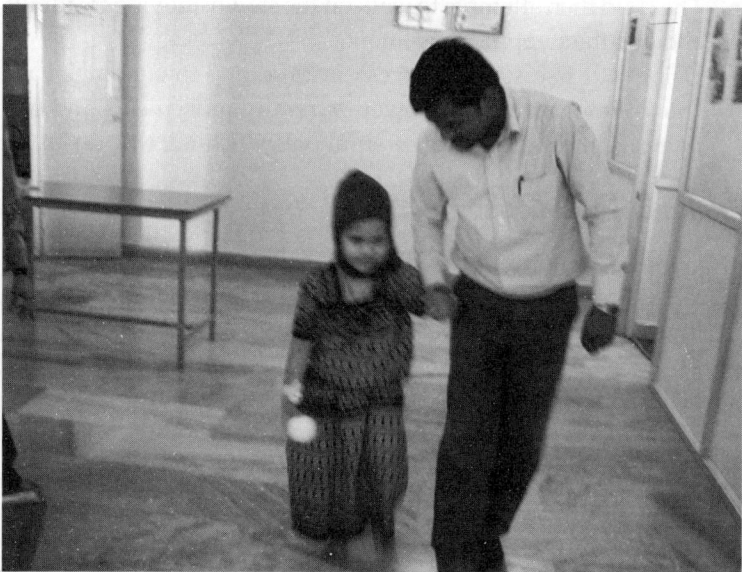

**Fig. 8.18:** Gait training

### Electrical Stimulation (ES)

- Electrical stimulation goal is to increase muscle strength and motor function
- Functional electrical stimulation (FES): The application of electrical stimulation during a given task or activity when a specific muscle is expected to be contracting
- Threshold electrical stimulation (TES): It is applied transcutaneously, is of low intensity, and does not elicit actual muscle contraction. TES is used to increase the muscle blood flow and bulk
- ES is used in children more than 4 to 5 years of old with diplegic or hemiplegic cerebral palsy
- Each session of NMES from 15 to 30 minutes. For duration that ranges from 1 month to 1 year.

### Body Weight Support Treadmill Training (BWSTT)

- The child is supported in a harness on the treadmill in an upright posture limiting weight bearing
- The child then attempts to walk on the slowly moving treadmill, eliciting the stepping movements
- Using 3 to 4 sessions per weak lasting for 3 to 4 months have shown improvement in lower extremity movements and gait patterns in children with cerebral palsy (Schindl MR, 2000).

### Conductive Education (CE)

- Conductive education (CE) was developed by Peto in the 1940
- CE use repeated verbal reinforcement to promote and facilitate intended motor activity by the child
- To develop independence in daily activities by the child by facilitating all aspects of child's development
- The child is encouraged to participate and practice all daily activities to the best of his/her abilities.

### Patterning

- The concept of patterning is based on theories developed by Fay, Delacto and, in the 1950 and 1960

Physical Therapy in Cerebral Palsy

- Motor development can be facilitated in the brain injured children by passively repeating the sequential steps of typical development, a process called patterning.

## Hippotherapy (HT)

- To improve muscle tone, balance and postural control.

## Acupuncture

- To reduce painful muscle spasms and overall motor function (Shi B, Bu H and Lin L, 1992).

## Hyperbaric Oxygen Therapy (HBOT)

- Use of HBOT is to increase the $O_2$ available to the neurons surrounding the injured area of the brain and revive those dormant neurons
- HBOT is to decrease brain edema by inducing cerebral vasoconstriction.

## Constraint-induced Therapy (CIT)

- CIT is to improve the use of affected upper extremity in a child hemiplegic cerebral palsy
- The normally functioning or stronger upper extremity is immobilized for a variable duration in order to force the use of the affected or weaker upper extremity over time
- The efficacy of this approach has not been estabilized and adverse effects of prolonged immobilization of the normally developing upper extremity are a significant concern (Echols, K, et.al 2002).

## Vojta Method

- The persistence of these newborn reflex patterns in a child with cerebral palsy interferes with postural development
- Facilitating the development of reflex locomotion.

## BIBLIOGRAPHY

- Butler C, Darrah J. Effects of neuro developmental treatment (NDT) for cerebral palsy: an AACPDM evidence report. Dev Med Child Neurol; 2001;43:778-90.
- Dali C, Hansen FJ, Pedersen SA, et al. Thershold electrical stimulation in ambulant children with cerebral palsy: a randomized double-based placbocontrolled clinical trial. Dev Med Child Neuro; 2002;44:364-69.
- Dilip R Patel. Therapeutic Interventions in cerebral palsy; symposium on Developmental and behavioral disorders II. Indian J Pediatric, 2005; 72(11): 979-89.
- Koman LA, Smith BP, Shilt JS. Cerebral palsy. Lancet, 2004;363:1619-31.
- Kliegman, Behrman, Jenson, Stanton. Nelson Text Book of Pediatrics; Cerebral palsy, 18th ed, Elsevier, 2008; 2: 2494-8, 670.
- Kliegman, Greenbanm Lye. Practical strategies in Pediatric Diagnosis and Therapy. 2nd ed, Elsevier, Philadelphia, 2004; p. 651.
- Kerr C, Mc Dowell B, McDonough S. Electrical stimulation in cerebral palsy; a review of effects on strength and motor function. Dev Med Child Neurol, 2004;46:205-13.
- Mayston M. Physical Therapy management of cerebral palsy; an update on treatment approaches, clinics in developmental medicine; 2004; 161:147-60.
- Meregillano G. Hippotherapy. Phys Med Rehabil clin N Am 2004; 15(14):843 -54.
- Schaaf R, Miller LJ. Occupational Therapy using a sensory integration approach for children with developmental disabilities, research reviews, 2005;11:143-8.
- Schindl MR, Forstner C, Kern H, et al. Treadmill training with partial body weight support in nonambulant patients with cerebral palsy. Arch Phys Med Rehabil 2000;81:301-06.
- Terence Stephon, Hamish W, Angela T. Clinical Paediatrics for Postgraduate Examinations, 3rd; Churchill Livingstone, 2006; p. 125-88.
- Veenakalra, Menon, PSN. Diseases of Central Nervous System; Parthasarthy A, et al. IAP Text book of Pediatrics, Jaypee Brothers, 4th ed, 2009; p 444-99.
- William WH, Myron JL, et al. Current diagnosis and treatment pediatrics; Cerebral palsy, 18th ed; McGraw Hill, USA, 2007; 771-82.

Physical Therapy in Cerebral Palsy

# Chapter

///////////////////////////////////

## 9

# Physical Therapy in Cerebellar Ataxia

## CEREBELLAR ATAXIA

- Cerebellar ataxia is a result of damage to the cerebellum or parts of the brain that connect to the cerebellum. This includes cerebellar peduncles and the pons, and red nucleus
- Cerebellar ataxia refers to a condition of unsteadiness of gait. Ataxia can result of damage to the cerebellum ( cerebellar ataxia) or posterior coloums of the spinal cord (sensory ataxia) or dysfunction of the vestibular system ( vestibular ataxia).

### Epidemiology

- Estimated prevalence: One in 12,500 adults with autosomal dominant cerebellar ataxia in the north east England
- Estimated minimum prevalence 10.2 in 100,000 people with late onset of cerebellar ataxia in south wales.

### Etiology

- Vascular
- Traumatic
- Developmental
- Neoplastic/Paraneoplastic
- Infections
- Inflammatory (e.g. Multiple sclerosis)
- Metabolic
- Toxic/drug-related (e.g. Alcohol)
- Epilepsy (In children).

### Clinical Manifestations

- Incoordination and unsteadiness (Figs 9.2A and B)
- Clumsiness
- Nystagmus
- Ataxia gait and in extreme cases impaired sitting balance (Fig. 9.1)
- Intention tremor
- Dysmetria or past-pointing – difficulty in controlling the termination of movements
- Dysdiadochokinesis – difficulty performing rapid alternating movements

- Dysarthria – slurred speech and slow with prolonged syllables (Scanning speech)
- Hypotonia – diminished resistance to passive movement
- Rebound phenomenon
- Contractures
- Dystonia
- Fatigue
- Bladder problems
- Sexual dysfunction
- Depression and other psychiatric symptoms
- Diplopia
- Pain (neuropathic).

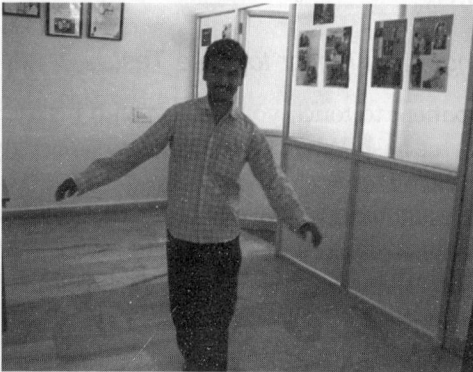

**Fig. 9.1:** Ataxic gait

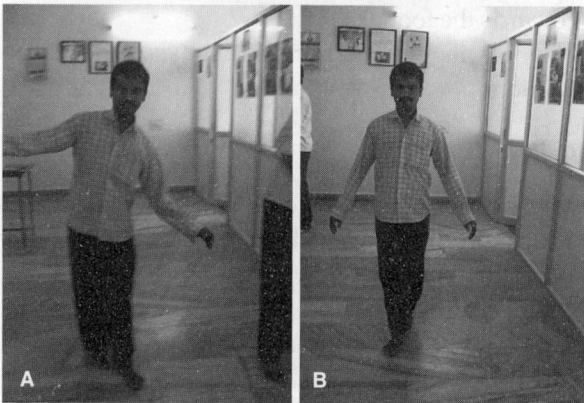

**Figs 9.2 A and B:** Unsteadiness and short step walking

## Diagnostic Investigations

- Creatinine, liver enzymes, electrophoresis, ESR, CRP, TFT, Vitamin $B_{12}$, fiolate, cholestrol, FBC.
- MRI of the brain
- Lumbar puncture
- Genetic tests
- EMG
- EEG.

## Assessment

- The assessment of ataxia should be integrated into a functional analysis were:

### Finger to Finger and Finger to Nose Tests

- Ask the patient to touch your finger with his/her finger and then touch his nose. When he has done this correctly ask him to repeat this faster
- The tester usually notes characteristics such as time taken and presence or absence of dysmetria and tremor.

### Heel-to-shin Test

- Patient is supine lying, and to place the heel of one leg on to the shin of the other, near the knee, then to slide the heel down the shin towards the foot
- Difficulty placing the heel because the dysmetric component of dysfunction.

### Romberg Test

- The test is performed in standing position. Patient is asked to stand still with arms stretched forward at shoulder height, with eyes open then closed
- Test for measuring ataxia
- Romberg sign can be using a force plate to measure of foot pressure (Black, et al. 1982).

Physical Therapy in Cerebellar Ataxia

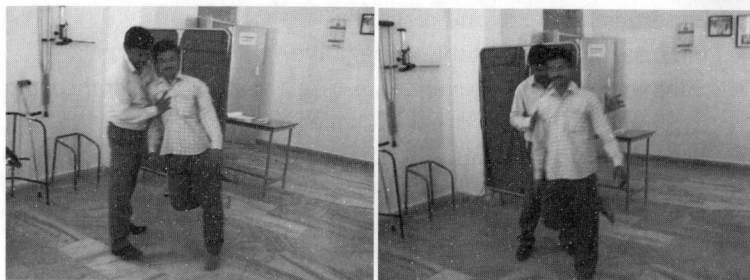

**Figs 9.3 and 9.4:** Romberg sign

## International Cooperative Ataxia Rating Scale (ICARS)

- This scale is measure of ataxia include: Finger to nose, heel to shin, walking, drawing, speech, oculomotor movement tests.

## Fahn Tremor Rating scale

- Assess to intension tremor in the period of the finger to nose test
- Useful tool for assessing movement disorders in people with ataxia, multiple sclerosis.

## Physical Therapist Examination

- The examination should consists of a complete history, a systemic review, and the implementation of the best available tests and measures to describe a patients impairments and functional limitations.

## Tests and Measures

- Assess range of motion
- Muscle strength (MMT) for trunk muscles, upper and lower extremities, and pelvic muscles
- Cranial nerve tested– impairment of ocular movements, visual field and acuity deficits, hearing loss, dysarthria and dysphagia
- Sensory integrity – position sense, sensation of pain, temperature and light test, diminished distally
- Reflex integrity–reflexes are decreased or absence of lower DTR
- Tone scales

- Superficial reflexes and reactions
- Babinski sign– is positive or negative
- Submaximal graded exercise testing - measure endurance and cardiovascular responses
- Balance measurements—Functional reach test, timed up and go test, down stairs test, Friedreich ataxia rating scale
- Gait measure–speed, symmetry and level of independence.

## PHYSICAL THERAPY INTERVENTION

- Physical therapy usually focus on strategies and compensatory techniques for maintaining or improving a patient's ability to continue to participate in all environmental contexts for as long as possible
- The aim of physical therapy is to improve gait, balance and trunk control for people with ataxia. Reducing tremor and improving functional movements. To reduce joint movement complexity
- Patient education and family members about the effects of disease progression on function and life style, potential therapeutic interventions, and realistic expectations regarding those interventions
- PNF
- Frenkel's exercise
- Dynamic training of postural with task and activity focus
- Gait and balance training
- Strengthening exercises
- Flexibility
- Visually guided movements (finger-to- nose test)
- Manipulation of visual information and hand movements
- Cold therapy–to decrease in muscle spindle, reduction in response of the long latency tone stretch reflex, decrease in nerve conduction velocity
- Wrist weighting–to reduce upper limb tremor
- Fitness training
- Mobility aids–light touch as a balance aid may be helpful for postural orientation and stability.

## OCCUPATIONAL THERAPY

- Occupational therapy is important intervention for patients with progressive neurological conditions in neurological conditions in maintaining independence and quality of life and to enable people to participate in self care
- Conservation energy technique
- Self care and toileting– encourage to bath or shower and consider providing seating with support for the back and arms
- Use thermoregulation devices on taps
- Bed, chair and toilet transfers
- Indoor mobility–use of walking aids in the home and other environments
- Use of walking frames may need to be reconsidered in very small areas
- Falls prevention.

## SPEECH AND LANGUAGE THERAPY

- The progressive ataxia may affect communication and or swallowing function
- *Dysphagia treatment:*
  - Use of oral muscle strengthening exercises
  - Use of the shaker exercise.

## BIBLIOGRAPHY

- Ataxia UK. Management of the Ataxias towards Best Clinical Practice, 2009.
- Fuller G. Neurological Examination Made Easy. 3rd ed, Churchill Livingstone, 2005.
- Gill B. et al. Rehabilitation of balance in two patients with cerebellar dysfunction, Phys Ther, 1999;77(5): 534-52.
- Gillen G. Improving mobility and community access in an adult with ataxia; A Case study. Am J Occup Ther, 2002;56:462-6.
- IIg.W, Syonfzik M, Brotz D, Burkand S, Giese MA, Scholes L. Intensive coordinate training improves motor performances in degenerative cerebellar disease.
- Jeka JJ. Light touch contact as a balance aid, Phys Ther, 1997; 77(5): 476-87.

- Maring JR, Croarkin E. Presentation and progression of Friedreich ataxia and implications for Physical therapist examination. Phys ther, 2007; 87(12): 1687-96.
- Michaael O, Harris. Rehabilitation management of Friedreich ataxia: Lower extremity force-control variability and gait performances. Neuro Rehabilitation and Neural repair, 2004;18(2): 117-24.
- Martin, et al. Effectiveness of Physiotherapy for adults with cerebellar dysfunction; a systemic Review. Clinical rehab, 2009;23:15-26.
- McGruder, et al. Weighted wrist cuffs or tremor reduction during eating in adults with static brain leasions. Am J Occupational Ther, 2003;57: 507-16.
- Schmitz Hubsuch et.al. Scale for the Assessment and rating of ataxia; Development of a new clinical scale, Neurology, 2006; 66(11): 1717-20.
- Vaz, et al. Treadmill training for ataxic patients; A single subject experimental design. Clinical rehab, 2008;22 (8):234-41.

# Chapter

////////////////////////////////////

## ⑩

# Orthotics in Neurorehabilitation

## ORTHOTICS

- Orthotics is a passive external device that support loads or assist or restrict relative motion between body segments. The word orthotics is derived from Greek for making or setting straight, and is a general term that encompasses bracing and splints. Orthotics or Orthoses plays an important role in the rehabilitation of patients with motor impairments. Orthotics include devices for the neck, upper limb, trunk and lower limb that are designed to guide motion, bear weight align body structures, protect joints or correct deformities. Orthoses are designed to work in co-operation with the intact body, and either control or assist movement. (Selzer, Clarke et al, 2003)

### Common Types of Orthoses

### Lower Limb Orthoses

*Foot Orthoses (FO)*

- Shoe inserts for correcting ankle and foot deformities.

*Ankle Foot Orthoses (AFO)*

- Short leg brace
- Commonly prescribed for weakness or paralysis of ankle dorsiflexion, inversion and eversion
- Prevent the patient from tripling secondary to weak or absent dorsi flexors
- L- Shaped brace typically made out of plastic
- Used patients with traumatic brain injury (TBI), spinal cord injury (SCI), and peripheral nerve injury
- Types: Metal, leather, plastic, and laminated
- To correct deformities of equinovalgus and equinovarus ankle foot deformities.

*Knee Ankle Foot Orthoses (KAFO)*

- Long leg brace
- Consists of proximal and distal thigh cuffs, calf band, double uprights with mechanical knee joints, and adjustable ankle joints

- KAFOs are commonly used for conditions caused by upper and lower motor neurone lesions
- Prescribed for knee stability and lower extremity weakness
- Stabilizes the knee and ankle
- Brace may be metal or plastic.

## Full Length Knee Ankle Foot Orthosis ( HKAFO)

- For stabilizing standing and gait stability
- To maintain upright posture and for standing stability
- Several HKAFO have been developed as Paralytic walking systems (Miller, 1997)
- The first is the Hip guidence orthosis (HGO) that locks the knee joint but has freely moving hip/ankle joints (Major et al 1981, Butler, et al, 1984)
- HKAFOs control hip flexion, extension, abduction, and adduction, rotation is controlled via foot plate.

## Trunk Orthosis

### Scott-Craig Orthosis

- A metal knee ankle foot orthosis (KAFO) used by spinal cord injury patients.

### Halo Orthosis

- An external brace designed to stabilize the cervical vertebrae.

### Four-Poster Orthosis

- Two plates (occipital and thoracic) with two anterior and two posterior posts to stabilize the head
- Used for moderate levels of control in indivials with cervical fracture/spinal cord injury.

### Jewett Orthosis

- An external method of providing stabilization to the thoracic and lumbar vertebrae

- Prevents hyper extension
- Three points of pressure on the sternum, lumbar spine and symphysis pubis.

### Thoracolumbosacral Orhosis (TLSO)

- For correcting scoliosis
- Any orthosis that provides external immobilization of the thoracic and lumbar spine.

### Lumabosacral Orthosis (LSO)

- For stabilizing low back fractures, elastic trunk support for preventing back injuries during lifting.

### Knight-Taylor Brace

- A method of applying external stabilization to the thoracic and lumbar vertebrae
- Typically utilized for fractures above the L3- region.

### Cervical Spine Orthosis (CO)

- Neck Braces for whiplash injuries or muscle spasm.

### Sterno Occipital Mandibular Immobilzation (SOMI) Brace

- A method of external stabilization for the cervical vertebrae.

### Reciprocating Gait Orthosis (RGO)

- Reciprocating gait orthosis (RGO) that links opposite joints so that extension of the hip on one side leads to flexion on the contra lateral side (Jefferson and Whittle 1990), e.g. spinal cord injury.

## Upper Limb Orthosis

### Shoulder and Elbow slings

- Weight support
- Prevents subluxation of stroke patients.

Orthotics in Neurorehabilitation

### Air Plane Splint

- Positions the patient's arm about 90 degree abduction, the elbow is flexed to 90 degree; the weight of the outstretched arm is borne on a padded lateral trunk bar and iliac crest band
- Used to immobilize the shoulder following injury of brachial plexus, e.g. Erb's Palsy, burns.

### Balanced Forearm Orthosis

- For feeding assist.

### Wrist Hand Orthoses

- To position the joints or assist in activities of daily living.

### Resting Splint (Cock-up-Splint)

- Wrist can be held in neutral or in 12 to 20 degree wrist extension
- Fingers supported, all phalanges slightly flexed with thumb in partial opposition and abduction
- Used for patients with stroke with paralysis, radial nerve injury, carpel tunnel syndrome, etc.

### Wrist-driven Prehension Orthosis

- Assists the patient in using wrist extensors to approximate the thumb and forefingers (Grip) in the absence of active finger's flexion, e.g. facilitates tenodesis grasp in the patient with Quadriplegia.

### Hand Orthoses

- To provide elastic resistance to finger extension, thus enhancing a strengthening program following stroke.

### Functional Electrical Stimulation Orthosis (FESO)

- FES was introduced by Liberson and coworkers and was applied to the peroneal nerve in the area of the fibular neck to produce dorsiflexion and eversion during the swing phase of gait

**Orthotics in Neurorehabilitation**

- Orthosis use and functional ambulation is facilitated by addition of electrical stimulation to specific muscles
- The pattern and sequence of muscle activation by portable stimulators is controlled by an externally worn miniaturized computer pack
- FES has been used in hemiparetic patients in an attempt to replace the AFO
- Requires PROM. good functional endurance
- In limited use with individuals with paraplegia–drop foot and scoliosis.
- The system worked best for gait problems by foot drop.

## BIBLIOGRAPHY

- Biering SF, Ryde H, Bojscn MF, Lyquist E. Shock absorbing material on the shoes of long leg braces for paraplegic walking. Prosthet orthot Int., 1990;14:27-32.
- Braddom RL. Physcial Medicine and Rehabilitation, 3rd ed. Philadelphia, WB. Saunders, 2007; p. 325-42.
- Cusick B, Sussman MD. Short Leg Casts; their role in the management of Cerebral palsy. Physcial and Occupational Ther in pediatric, 1982; 2:93-110.
- Fess EE. Hand and upper extremity Splinting: Principles and Methods, 3rd ed, St.Louis, Mosby, 2004; p. 37-41.
- Goldberg B, Hsu JD. Atlas of Orthosis and Assistive Devices, 3rd ed. St.Louis, Mosby, 1997.
- Hebert JS, Liggins AB. Gait Evaluation of an automatic stance -control Knee Orthosis in a patient with Postpolio myelitis. Arch Phys Med Rehabil; 2005;86(8):1676-80.
- Johnson RM,Hart DL, Simmons EF, et al. Cervical Orthosis: A study comparing their effectiveness in restricting cervical motion in normal subjects. J Bone Joint Surg (Am); 1997; p. 59-332.
- King S. The immediate and short term effects of a Wrist Extension Orthosis on Upper - extremity kinematics and range of shoulder motion, Am J Occup Ther 2003;57: p. 517-24, .
- Lehmann JF. Biomechanics of Ankle Foot Orthosis: prescription and Design, Arch Phys Med Rehabil, 1979;60:200-7.
- Lusardi MM, Nielsen CC. Orthotics and Prosthetics in Rehabilitation. Boston, Butterworth Heinemann, 2000.
- Lysell E. Motion in the Cervical Spine, thesis. Act Orthop Scand suppl, 1969;123.

Orthotics in Neurorehabilitation

- Nawoczenski D, Epler M. Orthotics in functional rehabilitation of the Lower limb. Philadelphia; WB, Saunders Co, 1997.
- Maiman D, Millington P, Novak S, et al. The Effects of the Thermoplastic Minerva body jacket or Cervical Spine Motion. Neurosurgey, 1989;25:363-68.
- Mckee P, Morgan L. Orthotics in Rehabiliation: Splinting the hand and body. Philadelphia, FA. Davis, 1998; p 1-17.
- Merati G, Sarchi P, Ferrarin M, et al. Paraplegic adaptation to assisted walking: Energy expenditure during wheelchair versus orthosis use. Spinal cord, 1979;38(1):37-44.
- Miller A, Temple T, Miller F. Impact of orthosis on the rate of scoliosis progression in children in children with Cerebral palsy, J Pediatric Orthop, 1996;16: 332-5.
- Morris C. A review of the efficacy of Lower limb Orthosis used for Cerebral palsy. Dev Med Child Neurol, 2002;44:205-11.
- Pope PM. Postural management and special seating. In: Edwards S, ed. Neurological Physiotherapy: A problem solving approach. 2nd ed, London; Churchil Livingstone, 2002; p189-217.
- O' Sullivan S, Schmitz. Physical Rehabilitation Assessment and treatment, 4th ed, Philadelphia, FA Davis CO, 2001.
- Orthotics and Prosthetics: physicians Pocket guide. New York, Rehabilitation Designs of America, 1999.

# Appendices

## Measurement Tools in Neurological Physical Therapy

| GLASGOW COMA SCALE | |
| --- | --- |
| Domain | Score |
| **Eyes opening** | |
| Open spontaneously | 4 |
| Open verbal command | 3 |
| Open to pain | 2 |
| No response | 1 |
| **Best Motor Response** | |
| Follows simple commands | 6 |
| To painful stimulus | 5 |
| Localization pain (Pulls examiner's hand away) | 4 |
| Flexion-withdrawal (Pulls limb away) | 4 |
| Flexion-abnormal (Decorticate) | 3 |
| Extension | 2 |
| No response | 1 |
| **Best Verbal Response** | |
| Oriented and converses | 5 |
| Disoriented and converses | 4 |
| Inappropriate words | 3 |
| Incomprehensible sounds | 2 |
| No response | 1 |
| Total score | 3 -15 |

**Ref.:** Teasdale G and Jannett. B (1974) – Assessment of Coma and impaired consciousness. A practical scale, Lancet ii; 81-83.

Appendices

## AMERICAN SPINAL INJURY ASSOCIATION
## (ASIA) SCALE

- A = Complete: No motor or sensory function is preserved in the sacral segments S4-S5.
- B = Incomplete: Sensory but not motor function is preserved below the neurological level and Includes the sacral segments S4-S5.
- C = Incomplete: Motor function is preserved below the neurological level, and more than half of key muscles below the neurological level have a muscle grade less than 3.
- D = Incomplete: Motor function is preserved below the neurological level, and at least half of key muscles below the neurological level have a muscle grade or 3 or more.
- E = Normal: Motor and sensory function is normal.

## CLINICAL SYNDROMES

- Central cord
- Brown-Sequard
- Anterior cord
- Conus Medullaris
- Cauda Equina.

**Ref.:** Lin.V (2003) – Spinal Cord Injury Medicine: Principle and Practice, New York.

| MODIFIED RANKIN SCALE | |
| --- | --- |
| **Score** | **Description** |
| 0 | No symptoms. |
| 1 | No significant disability despite symptoms; able to carry out all duties and activities. |
| 2 | Slight disability; unable to carry out all previous activities but able to look after own affairs without assistance. |
| 3 | Moderate severe disability requiring some help but able to walk without assistance. |
| 4 | Moderate severe disability; unable to walk without assistance and unable to attend to own bodily needs without assistance. |
| 5 | Severe disability; bedridden, incontinent, and requiring constant nursing care and attention. |

**Ref.:** Rankin J. (1957)–Cerebral Vascular accidents in patient over the age of 60. Scott. Med. J; 2; 200-15.

Appendices

# APPENDIX: D

| RANCHO LOS AMIGOS SCALE (FOR LEVEL OF COGNITIVE FUNCTIONING) | |
|---|---|
| *Level* | *Response* |
| I | No response: Patient does not respond to external stimuli and appears asleep. |
| II | Generalized response: Patient reacts to external stimuli in non-specific, inconsistent<br>– And nonpurposeful manner with stereotypic and limited response. |
| III | Localized response: Patient response specifically and consistently with delays to stimuli but may follow simple commands for motor action. |
| IV | Confused, inappropritate, agitated response: Patients exhibits bizarre, nonpurposeful,<br>– Incoherent, or inappropriate behaviors; has no short-term recall; attention is short and<br>– Nonselective. |
| V | Confused, inappropriate, nonagitated response. Patient gives random, fragmented, and nonpurposeful responses to complex or unstructured stimuli. Simple commands are:<br>– Followed consistently, memory and selective attention are impaired and new information<br>Is not retained. |
| VI. | Confused, appropriate response: Patient gives context-appropriate, Goal directed<br>– Responses, dependent on external input for direction. There is carry over for relearned<br>– But not for new tasks, and recent memory problems persist. |
| VII. | Automatic, appropriate response: Patient behaves appropriately in familiar settings:<br>– Performs daily routines automatically, and shows carry over for new learning at lower than normal rates. Patient initiates social interactions, but judgments remains impaired. |
| VIII. | Purposeful, appropriate response: Patient is oriented and responds to the environment,<br>– But abstract reasoning abilities are decreased relative to premorbid levels. |

Ref.: Hagen C, Malkmus D, Durham P. (1979) – Levels of cognitive functioning. In Rehabilitation of the Head Injured Athlete. Downey, CA, Professional Staff Association of Rancho Los Amigos Hospital.

Appendices

| STATIC BALANCE SCALE | |
| --- | --- |
| Grade | Description |
| 0 | Unable to stand (i.e. worse than next grade). |
| 1 | Able to stand with feet apart, but less than 30 second. |
| 2 | Stand with feet apart for 30 second, but not with feet together. |
| 3 | Stand with feet together, but less than 30 second. |
| 4 | Stand feet together, 30 second or more. |

**Ref.:** Bohannon et.al (1993) – Ordinal and timed balance Measurements; reliability and validity in Parents with stroke, clinical Rehabilitation, 7; 9-13.

# INDEX